Doing It Well

WALKING THROUGH CANCER WITH HOPE

Joanne Schreuders

DOING IT WELL
Copyright © 2024 by Joanne Schreuders

Scriptures taken from the Holy Bible, New International Version®, NIV®. Copyright © 1973, 1978, 1984, 2011 by Biblica, Inc.™ Used by permission of Zondervan. All rights reserved worldwide. www.zondervan.com The "NIV" and "New International Version" are trademarks registered in the United States Patent and Trademark Office by Biblica, Inc.™

This material is not intended as a substitution for medical advice. Please consult a physician before undertaking any changes to diet, exercise, or medication.

Printed in Canada

ISBN: 978-1-4866-2548-2
eBook ISBN: 978-1-4866-2549-9

Word Alive Press
119 De Baets Street Winnipeg, MB R2J 3R9
www.wordalivepress.ca

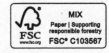

MIX
Paper | Supporting
responsible forestry
FSC
www.fsc.org   FSC® C103567

Cataloguing in Publication information can be obtained from Library and Archives Canada.

Contents

Introduction

"For I wrote you out of great distress and anguish of heart and with many tears, not to grieve you but to let you know the depth of my love for you."

—2 Corinthians 2:4

THIS STORY IS from my perspective, not from Jim's perspective or that of one of my ten children. They have their own stories to tell.

I tell you our story, not for sympathy, but to sympathize.

I tell you our story, not because I wanted this experience, but because we had this experience.

I tell you our story, so you can also know that all things are possible with Christ, even on the really hard days.

I tell you our story, hoping you can see the hope of Christ.

I would like to introduce you to Jim's family. His parents, Art and Corrie Schreuders, have four children.

     1. Julia married Henk and have eight children.

     2. Jim married Joanne and have ten children.

     3. Mary married Joe and have two children.

     4. Jonathan married Rio and have two children.

Jim and I, Joanne, have ten children. Yes, together.

     1. Derek married Danielle and have Chloe and Parker.

     2. Desiree married Joey and have Andrew, Eva and Peter.

     3. Nicolas married Jodi and have Allie and Graham (and Natalie)

     4. Nathan married Jessica and have Darius and Aria (and Mason)

     5. Victoria and her boyfriend (now husband) Seth.

6. Christina married Cody and have Wesley and Sophia
7. Elly
8. Melissa
9. Calvin
10. Joshua

These people will come in and out of the story along with other friends who I will introduce you to along the way.

Then there were Jim's awesome doctors:
- Dr. Thornton (family doctor and later palliative care doctor)
- Dr. Ferguson (cancer doctor)
- Dr. Fortin (lung surgeon)
- Dr. Lang (radiation doctor)
- Dr. Logan (drug/chemotherapy doctor)
- Dr. Palmer (radiation doctor)

And others behind the scenes that we never met.

But above all I want to thank Christ Jesus my Lord, who has given me (and Jim) strength to walk this path. Thank you for guiding me through the writing of this book and showing yourself to me in every step. May Your name be glorified now and forevermore. Amen.

What Is It?

"HON, FEEL THIS bump here?" Jim said as he put my hand on the outside of his upper right thigh. "You feel that? What do you think?"

It felt like a hard, inflamed muscle. "Yep, I feel it. Did you hit it on something?"

"Not that I can remember. When I do certain things, it gets uncomfortable. I've been wondering if I should see the doctor. It's just all this COVID stuff. Maybe I shouldn't."

"I've heard they are doing some visits over the phone now. So maybe just call and see if you can talk to Dr. Thornton?"

First, he had to ask his personal expert—his mom—for her diagnosis. Mom, a retired career nurse, also encouraged him to call the family doctor as she was not sure what it was either.

Life with our large family had come to a screeching halt due to the outbreak of COVID-19 during March Break in 2020. We were blessed, as Jim could still work at Premier Equipment in Tavistock because farm-related businesses were classified as essential. But there were no longer homeschool or church outings for our family. The only time I went out was to go to the grocery store once every week, occasionally twice if a second trip was completely necessary. There was fear in the air. When I walked into the grocery store, which provided shoppers with disposal gloves, the mask covering my mouth and nose caused my glasses to fog up. When I readjusted my glasses, I was shocked to see all the arrows on the grocery store floor; everyone was moving in the same direction. At the cashier there were stickers for you to stand on as a reminder to stay six feet apart from others.

In April, our daughter Christina's wedding date was drawing closer. She had the dress, the hall, and even the caterer all booked. They just needed to get a marriage license from the township. Sadly, she had to postpone her wedding because the township offices were shut down.

It was also around this time, having finished our dinner devotional book, that Melissa, seventeen, asked if we could just study a book of the Bible. She chose the book of Job. Asked why Job, she said it just came to mind, and she didn't know much about that one. Well, it was the best book for us to read during this time; there was no doubt in our minds. During the coming days, we could easily relate to Job. We learned it is okay to cry out to God and ask him why. But when you ask God why, you still have to trust in God's big plan for each of us, even though you cannot see his plan. *"Trust in the LORD with all your heart and lean not on your own understanding; in all your ways acknowledge him, and he will make your paths straight"* (Proverbs 3:5–6).

In April 2020, Jim called to book a phone visit with Dr. Thornton, our family doctor. After they chatted about the bump, she said she was pretty sure she knew what it was even though she hadn't seen it. He would have to come in person after picking up some steroids at the drugstore. At that time, she would inject them into his thigh, and this should make the bump disintegrate.

Taking the steroids with him, Jim entered Dr. Thornton's office alone as I was not allowed in.

"That is not what I thought it was," she said after taking one look at it. "I know what that is. I have two other patients with the same type of lump. We need to send you to a cancer doctor." She suggested a highly regarded doctor at Mount Sinai Hospital in Toronto. Jim agreed to go meet with this doctor before he came home to relate the discussion to me. I was shocked. Cancer? I felt in a haze. Do we talk about it? I decided I would follow his lead. I was mystified why his behaviour didn't seem to match the diagnosis. I couldn't believe how well Jim was taking this news.

Think about it.

Dr. Google can be a scary place. I didn't want to know. Much, much later, I learned that there are "safe" and helpful places to find answers. The Canadian Cancer Society website is one of those places that give the basic answers, as every cancer is as unique as the person. "Cancer isn't one disease but more than 100. And depending on how you classify cancer, you could even say that there are more than 200 types."[1]

---

[1] "What is Cancer?," Canadian Cancer Society, 2023, https://cancer.ca/en/cancer-information/what-is-cancer.

"Tumours are groups of abnormal cells that form lumps or growths. They can start in any one of the trillions of cells in our bodies. Tumours grow and behave differently depending on whether they are cancerous (malignant), non-cancerous (benign) or pre-cancerous." – Canadian Cancer Society.[2]

Before Christmas, and even before any talk of cancer, I started having thoughts about what I would do if Jim wasn't here. Could I care for this family on my own? At first, I was shocked at how vivid the thoughts were. I felt bad for having these thoughts, especially when I would answer yes, I believed I could care for this family, with God's help. I had read *War Room: Prayer Is a Powerful Weapon* by Chris Fabry.[3] What stood out for me was that we need to pray and get right with God *before* trouble comes our way. We can stand more firm with God if we have a strong relationship with him before unexpected events happen in our lives. I would sit and wonder what big event was coming. Life can't just move along peacefully, uneventfully—can it? And now I find myself reading *The Practice of the Presence of God* by Brother Lawrence[4]. This book has very short chapters on how Brother Lawrence prays continually, being one with God - all - the - time. Oh, how I want that, not getting frustrated at things big or small, seeing God in *everything* I do.

Now that I found out about Jim, I feel an odd sense of peace. God is here; He knows what is happening. If He calls Jim home, He will still be here. He won't leave me. So, I must cling to him (God), stay in his presence, and I will never be alone. When I think of myself and what I will miss out on, that's when I get sad. When I start to worry and begin to deal with things on my own, I am the one awake into the wee hours of the night thinking. But if I let God take the reins and I come along for the ride, and oh, it will be a ride, I am in good hands. So, till then, I will take every day striving not to overreact to my kids' requests, whether simple or crazy, and strive to be in the presence of God first, loving my husband and kids second. The situation between us might change, but God is always there. He is constant. As Ralph Abernathy said, 'I don't know what the future may hold, but I know who holds the future.'

---

[2] "Types of Tumours," Canadian Cancer Society, 2023, https://cancer.ca/en/cancer-information/what-is-cancer/types-of-tumours.

[3] Chris Fabry, *War Room: Prayer Is a Powerful Weapon* (Carol Stream, Il: Tyndale House, 2015)

[4] Brother Lawrence, *The Practice of the Presence of God* (Whitaker House, 1982).

The Adventure Begins

MAY 28, 2020, arrived with the sun shining as Jim and I started for Mount Sinai Hospital. I knew I wouldn't be allowed into the hospital, as COVID was still a big part of life. But I was there for moral support, the two-hour drive, and another two hours back. I took a book to read and some slippers I was knitting in case I couldn't concentrate on the words in the book. We made plans on the drive that he would get me on a speaker call so I could hear what the doctor had to say.

As we made our way through downtown Toronto, Jim missed our exit and had to take the next one (Okay, maybe that was my fault). It felt strange as traffic was almost nonexistent. During the COVID pandemic, a bustling city like Toronto had *no one* outside. We could count the cars we saw on one hand. It was very eerie, reminding us of a ghost town from the movies—nothing we had ever experienced before.

After parking, we found a rare restaurant that was open near the hospital for us to use the restrooms. As the time of Jim's appointment crept closer, we made our way to the hospital. I kissed and hugged Jim at the hospital door while assuring him I would be praying. Slowly, I returned to the parking garage across the street. After taking the elevator up three floors, I climbed back into the truck with butterflies in my stomach. I prayed. I tried to read, but the words blurred as my mind tried reaching out to Jim through those thick concrete walls. Feeling useless, I prayed more. Jim texted me while he waited for his biopsy. Silence while he went through the painful procedure. Then he texted again as they tried squeezing him in for a CT scan. Thinking it would be a long wait, we were surprised how quick he was in and out. Now we had to wait for the doctor. Trying to keep it light, our texting took on a joking tone—then more silence. I waited, anticipating the call where I would be connected to the doctor's visit.

Catching movement in front of me as I knitted, I looked up to see Jim get off the parking garage elevator with a slight limp. I was shocked to see him. *What about talking to the doctor?* ran through my head. *I missed the doctor's diagnosis!* I was angry by the time he opened the door of the truck. Angry that he wouldn't let me in on the doctor's visit. I needed to know the truth. But then I wondered if he even saw the doctor since not much time had passed. Maybe he didn't? Oh, *I'm so confused and frustrated* I thought as he climbed into the truck beside me.

"I'm sorry, I didn't have time to call you," he said as I tried to calm myself and quietly listened. "He just came in and started talking. 'Mr. Schreuders, this is not the 80s, so you get to keep your leg.' That was the first thing he said. Apparently, it is the same cancer as Terry Fox." Jim proceeded to draw me the diagram on a napkin which the doctor had drawn for him, explaining that the cancer was a lump with tails running beside his leg muscle. This cancer was a soft tissue sarcoma cancer. Dr. Ferguson recommended radiation and then a few weeks off for the radiation to keep working, followed by surgery. On the way home, there were long moments of silence, both of us trying to let this new information sink in.

About forty minutes into the drive, Jim turned to me. With astonishment in his voice, he said into the stillness of the truck cab, "I have cancer!" He then admitted that he was expecting Dr. Ferguson to tell him that our family doctor was wrong and he didn't have cancer after all.

That night Jim posted in the FamJam our family group chat, "Hello, Dad bod here! So, I had my appointment today at Mount Sinai Hospital Toronto. Had a biopsy and CT scan to see if the cancer had spread, but I won't have the final results till later next week. In the meantime, they want me to get started on radiation treatments to treat the area around the tumour. They assured me this is very treatable and I should be around for a long time to come. Thanks for your prayers and concerns."

Jim knew he had to let his mom and dad know. But telling his mom would break her heart. He put on his best puppy dog eyes and asked me to please tell his mom. My laughter took him by surprise as he was earnest about his request.

"What's so funny?" he asked.

"I just remember when I had my tumour, and you told me I had to call and tell my parents. I distinctly remember you telling me that *I* had to do it. You would not do it for me."

Looking at his feet, "I know, I'm a chicken." Then, looking up, he reminded me, "But it's my mom. I'm her son!"

Sighing deeply and taking a minute to contemplate, I said, "Even though I think you should tell them for making me tell mine, I remember how hard it was to call my parents. So, I will agree to call your parents." He was very grateful.

Being a mother myself, I knew how hard it was for her to hear what I had to tell her; her son had cancer. I knew right from the beginning that, being a retired nurse in the surgical unit, she would know more than we would about any surgeries and such.

She would know what questions to ask. She would also know what the answers would mean. My heart went out to her, and her son.

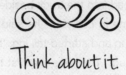

Think about it

This might not have been a path you would have chosen for yourself, but know that our faith is tested in the difficult and mundane things of life. What would change if you looked at them as opportunities to test, strengthen, and perfect your life with Christ? A path leading to a deeper, unbeatable, unbelievable joy? *"Not only so, but we also rejoice in our sufferings, because we know that suffering produces perseverance; perseverance, character; and character, hope. And hope does not disappoint us, because God has poured out his love into our hearts by the Holy Spirit, whom he has given us"* (Romans 5:3–5).

Our pastor, Pastor Martin, asked if he could visit after Jim gave him a brief outline of what was happening in our lives. Sitting out on the front porch, later that week, each with a cold glass of water in hand, Jim explained what had happened since April, and concluded with what the doctor had suggested for the upcoming days. Pastor Martin then asked Jim how he was handling all the news. Jim responded that we didn't know much yet, but that he was pretty optimistic about what the doctor told him, including the plan for treatment.

"And how are you doing with all of this Joanne?" he asked genuinely, turning to me. Slightly taken aback that he would ask me when this was about Jim, I cautiously looked at Jim. Inside I struggled with what to tell him. Do I tell him how I am feeling? Jim and I had talked about it. It wouldn't be a surprise.

I inhaled slowly, then cautiously turned back to the pastor and said, "I feel we need prayer, but Jim wants to keep it to ourselves now till we know more of what's going on. This is his story to tell, so I will respect him by not saying anything. But I disagree." Out of the corner of my eye, I could see Jim considering my words again. Pastor Martin understood Jim's concerns—some people might just use it as gossip—but he also agreed with me, suggesting to Jim that maybe he could tell only a select few close friends. After a pleasant visit, he left our porch heading for home, and Jim and I continued talking. Jim realized that I, being a woman, needed to share; I needed to have people praying for us. Whereas Jim, being a guy, didn't feel the need to talk about it. He agreed to let me tell three friends of his choosing. It didn't go unnoticed by me that these friends lived over an hour from us. These friends would have no way of telling others who lived close by or those in our church family.

As time for the radiation treatment grew closer, Jim felt the need for prayer also, finally allowing the Pastor to let our church family know. This was when a specific prayer request list was started for family and close friends, which lengthened as time went on. It included those who we knew were serious about praying for us.

Think about it

God made us all unique, and our paths in life are unique. We each process things differently. Some of us talk it through with others, while others quietly process in our own minds. But each of us needs time to process with God, away from others. Are you getting that time alone? Are you giving someone you love that time alone? We each need this time; it is very important to our relationship with God. During this time, it is okay to cry out to God as David did in Psalm 57:1. *"Have mercy on me, my God, have mercy on me, for in you my soul takes refuge. I will take refuge in the shadow of your wings until the disaster has passed."*

As you continue in Psalm 57, you will notice that verses nine and ten give praise to the Lord as we also should do. *"I will praise you, Lord, among the nations; I will sing of you among the peoples. For great is your love, reaching to the heavens; your faithfulness reaches to the skies."*

Jim and I were at Dr. Thornton's office together for another concern, when she turned the conversation to Jim's cancer.

"Do you guys have your affairs in order?" she asked. Going on to imply this was going to be a wild ride. "I have two patients that have this same type of cancer. One has surgery every couple of years whenever another tumour shows up. She has been doing this for a handful of years now. Another patient has not had it long and is not doing well. So, I just want you to know that it could be a long time that Jim is off work. Or it might not be." This conversation was hard to swallow, but we were thankful for the warning.

Being the planner of us two, I started looking into our finances to see what we could do to prepare ourselves for no income or as little as unemployment insurance would provide for us. Could we pay our bills on unemployment insurance? One big bill, our mortgage, we were trying to pay off as soon as possible. I called the mortgage broker to explain our situation. They helped us by cutting our mortgage payments by sixty percent, but we were warned that this was a one-time deal; once we returned to the original payments, we couldn't do this again. Another payment was going into our retirement fund. We decided to also stop that one for now, agreeing to start it back up when we were sure Jim was well again. Feeling a bit better now that we were doing some "planning," I breathed a sigh of relief.

Think about it.

If you foresee financial struggles coming your way, consider calling the companies that hold your bills. Explain your situation to them and see what they have to offer you. You might be pleasantly surprised at what they can do to help.

The lifting of the restrictions and the opening of municipal buildings also brought thoughts of an upcoming wedding for Christina. What do we do?

"I want my dad to walk me down the aisle. So we have decided to wait until after his radiation and surgery, when he is walking again." She let everyone know. We also hoped that all the restrictions for large gatherings would be lifted by then, so we could have the wedding she always wanted.

One Friday night, just after we went to bed, the phone on Jim's side of the bed rang. I could hear the voice of one of my children, but I couldn't make out what they were saying.

"You sure you guys are okay?" asked Jim, going over where they were exactly.

"I'll get a chain and be right there," he said, swinging his legs out of bed. Then, hanging up the phone, he told me they had rolled their pickup truck going too fast through a corner on a back gravel road. It wasn't the first time we were called out of bed for something like this. But they knew to always start the conversation with, "We are fine."

I was concerned whether Jim would be able to maneuver around with his sore leg. Not only that, but cancer had started to take its toll on him, making him tire faster. Did he have the strength to be up late?

"I'll be fine," he assured me. "They need me." Again, we thanked the Lord that everyone was safe.

Once there, realizing the truck had rolled back onto its wheels and would still run, Jim needed to find two tires to replace the ones that blew. He made a quick call to our oldest son Derek whom he knew had a truck in his farmyard with the same tires. Derek arrived, helping to get the truck back on the road so Jim could drive the roof-wrinkled truck—minus the back windows—home. The shaking child had to get behind the wheel of Dad's truck and drive it home. Yet another life lesson learned the hard way.

Jim didn't know what life would look like with radiation treatments, so he didn't know how to tell his boss. You see, Jim used to work in Listowel as a salesperson for Premiere. His present boss had worked hard to get Jim transferred to the parts department in Tavistock. After three intense meetings, Jim finally agreed to the move this past January, in part so that he would be closer to his aging parents. But how would he tell his boss that he would need an unknown number of days off?

Jim booked an appointment to speak with him one Monday morning. Nervously, Jim entered the boss's office. Taking a seat, he began the conversation with pleasantries. After this, Jim briefly summarized the cancer he had and that he would need radiation treatment. Then, with care and understanding, the boss told Jim about his own lung cancer and what he had been through and was still going through. Relief washed over Jim as he knew God had put him in Tavistock for just a time as this. That night, when Jim came home after work, he told me he went into that meeting thinking he would be the one talking, but instead, he listened. Knowing that someone understood, relief washed over him; it was so freeing. His boss knew Jim wouldn't take advantage of the situation. He warned Jim that if he was too tired, he needed to go home and rest; if he had an appointment or an emergency, he should just go. Both of us thanked the Lord for this understanding gentleman in our lives.

Jim often told me, "I want to do this well." He wanted to keep a positive outlook and show God's love through it all. The way he did this was by not dwelling on his circumstances, and continuing to be himself. Known for joking around, he continued this with those he encountered in his everyday life.

The Listowel Premier office, where Jim used to work, and the Tavistock Premier office, where he now worked, sometimes had parts on the other store's shelves that they needed. It wasn't uncommon to open a large box to find a smaller box containing yet another even smaller box inside before finding the part that was needed. Or a transfer might be a large box full of bubble wrap with an extremely small part somewhere inside. These transfers were just one of the many ways that Jim would brighten up someone else's day.

Jim was also known for pulling harmless practical jokes on our kids to pass the time. One night he laid out the bubble wrap that he had brought home from work just inside the man door of the garage. Late that night, when Melissa tried to come in silently, she was greeted with popping bubble wrap under her feet. She knew right away that Dad was up to his sneaky tricks, so she dragged it into the house with her, laying it outside our bedroom door for Dad to find when he got up in the morning.

The Next Step

WHILE JIM WENT to his consultation appointment in London, I knelt beside my bed, praying for Jim and waiting for the call to join the meeting. Once the doctor had me on the call, I took notes so we could remember the details. We were told radiation and surgery are the things that help for sarcoma cancers; chemo would only be a last resort as it does not work well on this type of cancer. During July and August of 2020, Jim was to have twenty-five radiation treatments on his leg. He could do the five days a week for five weeks at the University Hospital in London, eliminating a daily drive to Toronto. He was also relieved that they could book the treatments for the end of each day, so he could still go to work for most of the day. After our call, Jim was sent to get tattoos on his leg. These tiny dots, or markers, were to give the radiation machine a starting point as they mapped out his leg for the radiation work.

"Tattoos? Dad got tattoos?" The question came from multiple children. "After all these years of telling us we couldn't get tattoos, he goes and gets some himself," they laughed.

"Well, you can hardly see them, and they tell me they will fade with time." Jim felt he needed to justify.

Before Jim made it home, I had called our friend and neighbour, who had also had radiation, for any advice she may have for us. She confirmed that Jim would need cream to put on the site a few times a day to keep the skin hydrated and to help keep the burn from being so intense. Glaxal Base moisturizing cream worked best for her. She suggested he even start a few days before the radiation. So that is what we did.

Earlier in our marriage, Jim made sure I knew that my job was to care for the family. Whenever I would talk about getting a job on the side, he would say, "Caring for a large family is a full-time job. It involves preparing meals, getting people to and from where they need to be, and all the rest. Doing everything needed to save us money is your job." He knew that when the surgery came, he would be unable to work and bring in the full income our family needed. Needing to support his family is what kept him working as long as possible. Having heard about some grants for cancer patients, I called the cancer clinic. The lady informed me they would pay up to five hundred dollars, since we lived outside their shuttle service area. So, we applied. Jim's work colleagues also generously gave us gas cards for the daily drive back and forth. God used these people to provide what we needed.

Not knowing what radiation would look like, Jim took every chance he could to get out on his motorbike, a 1984 Yamaha Venture Royale. This was his happy place— where he could process his thoughts and pray. Whenever he could, he would drive his bike to work. After work, if it was nice weather, he would take one of the kids, or me, with him for, as he would say, "a ride around the block." We could count on being gone for an hour at least.

The plan was that Jim would drive the thirty minutes to work in Tavistock, be there a little after 7:00 am, and work the parts counter until about 4:00 pm. From there, he took the fifty-minute drive to University Hospital for his treatment which would take about fifteen minutes. Then, when that was finished, he would make the forty-minute drive back home. He was doing well the first couple of weeks. He was only a little tired and had no signs of a radiation burn on his leg.

Jim's birthday arrived in the middle of his treatments. I wanted to get him something special, something he wouldn't go out and buy himself. I came up with a plan. On the Saturday morning of his birthday, I suggested a motorcycle trip to St. Jacobs, knowing he wouldn't object to a motorcycle ride. Once we arrived, we walked around as I tried to find the gift at an outside booth. But the more I looked the more disappointed I became, unable to find that special gift I had in mind.

"What are you looking for?" he asked, seeing that I was distracted.

"Your birthday gift. It used to be in a booth right here, but now they aren't," I sadly told him.

"Well, what was it?" he asked. Seeing no hope, but to tell him my idea, I sighed.

"I was going to get you one of those wind chimes you like so much."

"You're right; they were here," he confirmed. "Maybe ask the lady over there." After inquiring, she said that we had the correct booth, but they were now at their other booth inside. After receiving directions, we headed indoors. Relieved to have found what I was looking for, we tried different ones out. Finally, finding the perfect one for us, I paid for the chimes, and we headed to the parking lot. As we approached the motorcycle, Jim stopped and turned to me.

"How are we going to get these chimes home?" he said, nodding down at the almost four-foot-long box in his hands, the length of the longest chime.

"Where is your sense of adventure, Mr. Schreuders?" I said with a smirk on my face. I climbed onto the motorbike, motioning for him to hand them to me. "I'll hold them between us."

"Crazy woman," he said, shaking his head as he handed me the chimes.

"I had a good teacher," I laughed. Well, we had a crazy drive home as the wind would catch the flat side of the box on the left or the right. Nevertheless, it was a good workout for me to keep hold of it on my lap and try to stay balanced while not pulling Jim off balance. At one point, I leaned ahead and said, "Too bad I can't hold it flat like airplane wings between us. Maybe we could fly!"

Once home, we hung up our treasure on the front porch. This made Jim's special outdoor spot much more enjoyable as the chimes sounded like church bells.

As the days of radiation turned into weeks, treatment started taking its toll on Jim. Did I mention that one of the side effects of cancer is being tired, which is also one of the side effects of radiation? After a full day of work and radiation treatment at night, he would have a small meal and then crash on his La-Z-Boy reclining chair. By 9:00 pm, I would tuck him into bed to do it again the next day. Once he completed half of the treatments, seeing how tired he was, I offered to have one of the kids drive me to his work at 4:00 pm daily, so I could drive him. But due to rising gas prices, he only took me up on it twice. He wanted to do this on his own. The two times I did drive him in, he slept the whole way there and home. This made me more nervous on the other days when he didn't let me drive him.

Laughter Is the Best Medicine

THURSDAY, SEPTEMBER 3, 2020. Jim drove the two of us to Mount Sinai in Toronto for Jim's pre-admit. Once finished, they told him he needed to come back on Sunday for his COVID test.

"You can't do that now?" he questioned.

"No sir, it has to be 48 hours before your surgery," they informed him.

"You have to be kidding me! You want me to drive four hours for a COVID test? Can't I get a test closer to home, and the results get sent here?"

"Sorry, sir. They only accept the tests done here where we are doing the surgery."

"Oh, for Pete's sake. This is just getting out of hand."

"Sorry, Sir."

It was then arranged that I would take the kids to church Sunday, and Derek would accompany Jim to Toronto for his COVID test. Spending one-on-one time with his oldest son was a rare treat, each having families of their own to care for. Upon their return, Jim said it all worked out well as they had forgotten some blood work on Thursday, and he could do that too while he was there.

Tuesday, September 7, Jim drove the two of us in the comfort of his Ford F150 crew cab pickup back to Toronto to arrive at 6:00 am. With little difficulty, we found the hotel I had located online, only a five-minute walk away from Mount Sinai Hospital. After struggling to find a parking place, as the pickup truck didn't fit in the underground parking garage, we gathered our stuff. Walking the short distance to the front lobby, I approached the manned registration counter.

"Can I please get a room for two nights? And I only need one bed."

"And what brings you to visit with us?" the kind gentleman asked.

"My husband is going for surgery."

"We have a special rate for those staying with us for medical reasons," he surprised us. I was already struggling with paying the cost of a hotel room I was not sharing with Jim.

Jim relieved me from this particular anxiety as we brought our luggage to my room, saying, "I am so glad you will be close to me and not back home. It just makes me feel so much better knowing you are here." Now I knew the cost didn't matter.

We knew that because of the COVID-19 pandemic, it was a gamble each day as to whether I would be allowed in the hospital to be with him. But we were willing to take that chance. With all our stuff left at the hotel, even Jim's phone and glasses, we walked hand in hand to the hospital. Jim and I agreed that I would bring his things tomorrow after surgery. With forced cheerfulness, tears in our eyes, and heavy hearts, we said, "See you tonight," while exchanging a kiss and a hug, both of us trying to be brave for the other. He turned and walked through the door, leaving me on the sidewalk. Tears escaped my eyelids and made a tiny river down my cheeks. I returned to the hotel room and tried not to look at anyone I passed. Once I got to my room, I felt lost, not knowing what to do now.

Having gone through the COVID screening questions, Jim made his way to the surgical unit. Once finished with all the prep work for the surgery, he sat. And sat. He looked around for magazines to read, but they had all been removed to keep the patients from contracting COVID. Realizing the grave error he had made by not taking his phone, he tried not to think about the coming hours. Time passed at an excruciatingly slow speed, making it feel like an eternity before they called his number at around 9:00 am.

His surgery took three hours. The surgeon called me at the hotel at 1:00 pm to let me know that everything went well. He informed me that someone would call and let me know when he was in his room so I could see him. I waited. I waited some more. I called the hospital to see if they had forgotten about me and if he was already in a regular room.

"No, he is still in recovery," came the reply. So, I tried to wait patiently while looking out the window at the tiny people and cars far below me. It was getting late; the sun was going down. Would I get in before visiting hours were over at 9:00 pm? I called back again a few hours later. They were still waiting for a bed to become available on the floor he needed to be on. Around 8:30 pm, I could finally talk with Jim personally on the phone as he was finally in his room. He was very groggy, slurring some of his words. I looked out my hotel window and saw that dusk had covered Toronto.

"Joanne, just stay there. I'm still really tired. Just come first thing in the morning," he advised. I was happy to oblige as I didn't like the thought of walking in downtown Toronto alone after dark. Standing at the window, as relief washed over me, I realized how tense I had been. I now looked—really looked—at the beautiful lights twinkling beyond my window. It did look pretty. I thanked God for the beauty before me and that Jim was okay. I prayed that he would have a good sleep with little pain.

The following day, I was at the hospital doors bright and early for the COVID screening. The lady looked at her watch. I knew she was taking note that it was fifteen minutes before official visiting hours. Would she let me in? I just needed to be with Jim. I needed to know he was okay. Looking up at me with a sly smile, she whispered, "Walk slowly." I smiled, thanking her.

Attempting to be slow, I found my way through the hospital to Jim. He looked really well and happy. No slurred speech or pain etching his face. But it didn't take long before I noticed a change in my husband. This man that I have loved for more than thirty-one years of marriage. This independent, strong man needed me, little, insignificant me. As if I was the strong leader and he was meekly following. Over and over, he said how much he needed me and wanted me to stay close. This was fine with me because I didn't want to leave his side either.

Jim told me with a sparkle in his eyes about trying to get out of bed and almost falling flat on his face because he couldn't feel his leg. He had forgotten that they had given him Demerol, a pain blocker, and put him out for surgery. He was feeling good!

Later in the day, the physiotherapist came to see how Jim was doing with his walking. During surgery, the surgeon had to remove some muscle with the tumour. Unfortunately, muscle does not grow back, so now he would have to learn to live without that muscle. With the help of his hospital walker, Jim hobbled to the door. After being reminded that he needed to put on his mask before entering the hall, the physiotherapist followed close behind. Jim went a little into the hall and she commented on how well he was doing. On his return to the room, coming past the bathroom, he wanted to try to go to the washroom again. Noticing a seat riser on the toilet, the therapist offered to remove it and get it out of the way for Jim. With the walker and Jim already in the bathroom, there was little room left to maneuver. So, being Jim, he lifted the walker and set it in the tub out of the way.

"Jim! You are supposed to be using that!" the therapist said in shock.

"Oh, right!" Jim snickered. Then we all laughed together.

We were relieved to be able to sit together all day except for Jim's short trip to get another X-ray. During that time, I went to grab dinner from the cooler and mini fridge in my hotel room. On my return, I stopped at the pharmacy in the hospital lobby. I looked through all the canes they had. "Maybe he wouldn't mind a bright blue one?" I thought with a smile. But, no, he would want a basic black one to not draw attention to himself. So, after purchasing the humdrum shiny black cane with the squishy handle, I returned to his room upstairs. Here, we enjoyed some quiet time together while sending messages to family and friends until Jim's old-fashioned telephone tone rang on his phone.

"How is it going, Dad? How are you feeling?" our twenty-six-year-old son, Nathan, cheerfully asked as he drove home from work. Jim gave a relatively upbeat reply as the pain blocker was wearing off, and he was getting slightly more uncomfortable. After talking for a few minutes, Nathan said he just had to make a quick stop and that he would call us back in a minute. So, we waited, but not too long, and we soon heard Jim's phone tone announcing Nathan's call.

"I'm back... (snicker, snicker)."

"Na-than," Jim said drawing his name out slowly and suspiciously. "What are you up to?"

"Oh, nothing. Hee hee."

We could hear that he was having difficulty keeping a straight face, "Nathan, we are your parents. We know you. Tell us what's up!"

Snickering, he replied, "I'm sure you will hear about it soon." He followed with a change of topic, of course. "So, how long will you need to be in the hospital, Dad?"

"A few days, Nate. Come on, tell us what's going on?"

"Patience, Dad. It should be coming on the FamJam soon. Well, gotta go now. (snicker) Love you, guys."

"Love you too."

With smiles, we tried to dream up what he was up to; we were unprepared for the picture on the FamJam just a few minutes later. There, on the phone screen, was a picture of a chicken. Well, not quite a full-grown chicken. You know, the in-between ugly stage of a chick and a chicken... in our shower! Scrawled across the top were the words, "Seriously, Nathan? What are we supposed to do with this!"

Having figured that his sisters would be at home "taking care of things" while mom and dad were in Toronto, Nathan wanted to test their ability to "care for things" like they claimed they could.

Jim laughed when he received a selfie of Nathan and the chicken in the shower. Nathan had taken the photo before sneaking out of the house. What he was not counting on was that Calvin had spied him as he passed Calvin's room on his quick and quiet retreat from the house.

"Dad, what do I do with this chicken now?" Our twenty-four-year-old daughter, Victoria, messaged.

"Feed it!" came Dad's cheeky reply.

You could hear the frustration in her text, "What do we feed the chicken, Dad?"

The kids went to the neighbour, our "adopted son," Lucas, who raised chickens, and asked for some chicken feed. We were later informed that the chicken's name would be Crispy.

"Oh no, Jim, they named the chicken; now we will have to keep it," Jim just smiled at me.

Think about it

Have you pulled a good, safe practical joke on anyone lately? Have you ever? Has anyone ever pulled one on you? Did you laugh? Are you snickering right now just thinking about it? Laughter reduces stress and revives your lungs, heart, and other muscles, on top of boosting your intake of oxygen. Did you know that fifteen minutes of laughter a day is equal to about two hours of sleep? So just laugh! *A cheerful heart is good medicine, but a crushed spirit dries up the bones*" (Proverbs 17:22).

During one of our very slow walks through the hallways, while discussing how to keep a chicken alive, we passed by the nurse's station. Having met Jim, it didn't take the nurses long to notice his fun-loving personality and quick wit. A nurse mentioned that she noticed that patients with upbeat, positive personalities heal faster and can go home sooner. At another pass by the nurse's station, another nurse felt comfortable enough to say to Jim, "Show off!" We then noticed that no one else was walking the halls. Jim was the only one. Why was no one else walking?

As we walked, we would stop to look at the artwork on the walls or read signs and pamphlets. One of these pamphlets told us that 11 South, the unit Jim was in, was a thirty-bed unit dealing with a rare type of cancer called sarcoma. "The sarcoma program at Mount Sinai Hospital is the largest multidisciplinary program of its type in Canada and allows patients to receive all of their cancer care needs on one unit." After reading this, we felt like we were in the right place. Another pamphlet made me stop to take a second look. It was titled, "Sex and Cancer." Of course, having ten children, this pamphlet piqued my interest. Our question was, "Why do they need to educate people about this?" We did notice some small but insignificant changes, but nothing to be concerned about. Little did we know.

Think about it.

The Canadian Cancer Society website has a booklet entitled *Sex, Intimacy and Cancer.* "Throughout the booklet, Canadians tell their stories. How cancer affected their sexuality and their ability to have sex. What they did about it and how they felt about it. Their stories can remind you that you are not alone and that help is available. Their experiences may be different from yours, but they remind us that sexual health is an important part of overall health—even when you have cancer."[5]

The next day, Jim convinced the doctors to let him go home. I wonder if it had to do with his whiteboard chart on the wall in his room. It said *(the italics is Jim's handwriting)*

> Expected date and time of discharge: *today*
> Activities: *Yoga*
> Precautions: *Handle with care*
> Special Instructions: *Rub his feet*
> Goals of the Day: *Home*
> Diet: *Pie, Pie, and more pie!*

Having been married to him for thirty years, his humour rubbed off on me, so I added below:

> Patient and Family Questions: *Can you send some extra pain meds home to give him when he meets the new boyfriend? (signed) Daughter*

Early that afternoon I was astounded when he was going to walk out of that hospital all on his own. The nurse and I finally convinced him to take a ride in the

---

[5] "Sex Intimacy and Cancer," Canadian Cancer Society, 2019, https://cancer.ca/en/cancer-information/resources/publications/sex-intimacy-and-cancer.

wheelchair to the hospital door, as he had no concept of how far it was. He struggled to bend his leg comfortably as he tried getting it on the footrest. Keeping it there was very uncomfortable for him as we went down from 11 South, into the elevator, and down the hall to the main doors at the back of the hospital. Having reached the doors and thankful to stretch out his leg again, he informed the nurse and me that he could walk to the truck and that I wouldn't need to bring the truck around. With the help of his cane and my arm, he made it across the street. We passed two parking garages and went up the elevator to the truck, just outside the third floor elevator doors. With relief, he settled into the passenger seat, trying hard to find a comfortable position with the extra pillows I had brought from home. I climbed in next to him in the driver's seat and exited the parking garage. I was dreading the Toronto traffic, but with Jim's directions, we made it with no issues.

After a quick stop at the New Hamburg McDonald's drive-thru to quiet my grumbling tummy, the discomfort started growing in his leg. Jim knew visiting his parents in Tavistock was out of the question. He decided to make a phone call to Mom instead, hoping to put her mind at ease. She was happy to hear all was well but still fretted over him, telling him to be careful and keep his leg up.

When we returned home, Jim went straight to his comfy recliner and sighed deeply. It was good to be home again. As per the nurse's instructions, Jim called the in-home nurse in Exeter. I was taken aback when I heard him tell the nurse he was well enough to drive into her office every few days. She would check the drainage tube sticking out of the bottom of his twelve-inch-long wound, ensuring it was still draining fluid from within and no infection was starting. He called his wound a caterpillar, as it bunched under the stitches. He struggled with how it looked even though the nurse and I told him it would flatten out after the stitches came out.

The evenings were challenging as we were used to snuggling. I didn't want to hurt Jim, so I stayed back, allowing room for the multiple pillows that he had around him to help prop his leg into a more comfortable position. After a few nights of this, he tried pulling me closer.

"Why are you so far away?" he asked. "I miss you."

"I don't want to hurt you," I said, hesitating but wanting to get closer.

"You won't hurt me," he reassured me, pulling me closer. "If I get uncomfortable, I promise I will let you know, okay?" Then, feeling more reassured, I snuggled in closer and a feeling of coming home came over me.

I was realizing that communication was the key, as we both struggled with what was happening in our relationship. Talking about it was a way we could help each other through the hard and awkward times.

On a Mission

ONE DAY, NOT even a week after returning home, he hobbled into the dining room.

"That probably was not a smart idea?" he said as I looked up from the school lesson I was checking. "I almost got stuck on my motorcycle."

"You did *what?*" I said, hoping I didn't hear him right. But I could see from his facial expression that I had. "Jim, the more you do, the more that vacuum will fill with fluid, and then you will have to have it in longer." I weakly reasoned as I knew he didn't like that vacuum tube at all. But he didn't fall for it. His drive to get better was to get back on that motorcycle. A few days later he put a tensor band around the tube on his leg so it wouldn't move, pulling his pants over it. He secured the vacuum in the front pocket of his John Deer hoodie. I was doing homeschool prep on the laptop when he came hobbling over to me at the dining room table. He leaned in from behind, kissing me on the cheek.

I whipped around as if stung, "No, you are *not* going on that motorcycle!" Slightly shocked, not knowing how I knew, he stared at me for a minute. Then a smirk climbed the corners of his mouth, his puppy dog eyes shone through, and he said in a childlike voice, "Awe come on, just a little one?" He is a grown man. This is what he lives for. What was I going to do to stop him?

"Please, please, please be careful!" I pleaded, and off he hobbled like a kid in a candy store.

The vacuum in his leg was still getting lots of fluid. We were told that sometimes fluid builds up because of the tube, but there is no way of knowing if the tube was a help or a hindrance. Their concern was not wanting to trap the fluid inside, or an infection could start.

The day came when it wasn't working correctly. The tube slowly started to make its way out of his leg, causing the vents to suck outside air instead of the fluid from within. Our nurse suggested we call his surgeon. So we did. However, we could only get as far as the receptionist, who was no help. I then drove him to our local hospital in St. Marys, where he was told to call the surgeon; they were not responsible for it. This vacuum was half in his leg and not working. He wanted it out so bad, and no one would deal with it. Advocating on Jim's behalf, his nurse in Exeter finally got through to the surgeon and received the okay to remove the vacuum. Once removed, the nurse put gentle pressure on his leg and squeezed fluid out of the hole at the bottom of his incision. Jim was intrigued, copying her pressure to watch more liquid come as she turned to get more gauze from the counter behind her. Turning back to see what he was doing, she reprimanded him, but he didn't care. He was just over the moon to be free from that vacuum.

His goal was to try to walk without a limp. Hobbling around the yard exercising his leg while Crispy followed was physio enough, so Jim didn't need to see a physiotherapist. Crispy was constantly close by pecking the ground around Jim for bugs or sitting in the shade under Jim's lawn chair. Those two seemed to do everything together, like a man and his dog. But this was a man and his chicken.

During this season, we would usually get up late Saturday mornings to find our son Nathan sitting on the front step with his son, Darius. After a long week of work it was his way of spending time with his son and letting his wife sleep in. On one of these early Saturday mornings, as we sat visiting, the weather grew warmer. Nathan pulled off Darius's sweater to reveal a white t-shirt with bold blue letters that said, "Big Brother." Jim and I were so excited to hear that our tenth grandchild was on the way! Two handfuls. We couldn't wait to share the news.

October arrived in all its fall glory, bringing with it cool air for our thirty-first wedding anniversary. We both wanted to go out and celebrate somehow but had to stay reasonably close to home, as sitting in a vehicle was still uncomfortable for Jim's leg. It was decided that we would attempt to go to Grand Bend and walk on the beach or sit on a bench while watching the water. Once there, it was not long till I noticed Jim was invigorated by the beach, his favourite spot in the world. He was heading toward the peer and then limping toward the lighthouse.

"Jim, the waves are big. We will get wet if we go to the end."

"Oh, come on, it will be fun!" he smiled, and I realized we wouldn't be returning to the truck dry. I watched as Jim hobbled on, hoping that if I stayed put, he would return to my side. But instead, he watched the waves, gauging his steps between the rhythm of the shallow water washing over the peer. He reached his goal of the light stand at the end of the pier but needed to climb up the light stand as the waves started to come higher and in more rapid succession. He tried to wave me over to him with his huge charming smile, but I was not taking the bait. This is when I could see from my end of the peer that he would struggle to get back. Was I willing to get wet also? Of course not! So, talking him through the waves that were now at his back, I took a movie on my phone. There had to be something I could use to show my kids what not to do. He tried to hobble at a fast pace toward me while I cringed, noticing this was very uncomfortable for him. "Stubborn man," I thought. Coming to the final stretch, he made a sudden unexpected maneuver. Seeing that a concrete berm to his left was higher, and could help him out of the water that was flowing deeper over the peer now, he took a painful hop-step up. Little did he know that the berm put him right in the path of a giant wave coming up alongside the peer. I yelled as he looked up, and the wave hit his pants from behind. Realizing he was already wet, he threw his hands up in the air and slowed his pace so he was more comfortable. Seeing that he was okay, just soggy, I let out a pent-up laugh, to which he joined in.

"That was cold!" he said once he had rejoined me.

"I'm sure it is. That's why I stayed here. Come on, let's get you in the warm truck."

Later at home, we enjoyed showing the kids the video I got of dad's adventure with the waves. I always admired how Jim was able to laugh at himself. He knew how to find fun in everyday things.

Think about it

Are you able to laugh at yourself? Are you able to enjoy your life? When life sends you an unexpected wave, do you get angry, or can you smile? *"So I commend the enjoyment of life, because nothing is better for a man under the sun than to eat and drink and be glad. Then joy will accompany him in his work all the days of the life God has given him under the sun"* (Ecclesiastes 8:15).

Wills

IT WAS TIME to look at our wills again. We noticed that the last will didn't include our four youngest children. So, we started the process by calling up Christian Stewardship Services. During a free video call, Hilco DeHaan went through the paperwork we had filled out beforehand. We had to make a few decisions about who were going to be the first and second executors of our estate and how our estate would be split. We had to decide at what age our children would acquire the funds from the estate. We had to assign guardians. Our younger children didn't know the guardians we had listed for our older children, so we had to search for new ones. This was not going to be easy. Who would know our boys, love them as we do, and raise them as we would like them to be raised, with our beliefs? Lots of prayers went into that. Hilco also discussed the need for a first and second for medical care decisions. These two people would be the spokespeople for decisions that needed to be made if we were both critically ill or in our case, if only one of us was left. Who would be okay with making the final decision and not regretting it later? We talked to the kids.

"Well, I can't decide on what colour to paint the walls, so I'm not your person," said one.

"Yeah, we already crossed you off the list," I said, laughing.

"It takes me two hours to pick a movie. It's not me," said another.

This made for long conversations as to what we wanted. How much pain or suffering would you endure to stay in this world? I told the kids, right off the bat, "I don't want to stay here. I want to be in heaven with my Lord! Don't put me on life support." Jim, on the other hand, always wanted to give the medical professionals every chance to keep him alive. He couldn't make that decision as quickly as I could. As I looked at him, my thoughts struggled. How can he not want to go? Is it really that hard of a decision? Well, apparently, it was for him. This non-decision was hard for me as he was putting me in a hard place. It was no longer a clear decision.

Think about it

Have you made your wills yet? Are they updated? Maybe you have your estate planning all in order, but what about your eternity planning? Have you read the paperwork, the Bible, and are you walking with Jesus, who will lead you to heaven to be with God? *"For God so loved the world that he gave his one and only Son, that whoever believes in him shall not perish but have eternal life"* (John 3:16).

Consider itemizing your possessions in a binder and listing who gets what. This can be extremely helpful for those who are left behind as they go through your estate. Why not give some of it away now? This can save much heartache and arguments later. *"Do not lay up for yourselves treasures on earth, where moth and rust destroy and where thieves break in and steal; but lay up for yourselves treasures in heaven, where neither moth nor rust destroys and where thieves do not break in and steal. For where your treasure is, there your heart will be also"* (Matthew 6:19–25).

Once all the paperwork was filled in, we had a meeting with all our children in the dining room. Sitting in a big circle, with the laptop on the bookshelf so Christina could join by video, we thanked all the kids for making this day work. We went through our wills and what was decided.

"In the event that you die, where do you want to be buried?" asked one. Jim and I looked at each other and smiled.

"I want to be buried in Fullarton and Dad in Avonton," I said.

"You guys don't want to be buried together?" came the shocked question.

"Yes, but we are still debating. I guess whoever goes last gets to decide!" We all laughed.

Being a frugal family, the discussion went on to, "We can just dig a hole in the backyard."

"The boys can build a pine box."

"Nowadays, you have to have a concrete vault."

"That's easy; I have access to a cement mixer." Knowing this was all in fun, we could all laugh together.

We ended the meeting by asking the kids to think about anything that they would like of ours and email a list. By doing this, we hoped to avoid any fights or arguments later. Once the requests started coming in, we were surprised to see what was important to each child. More surprising was that no two wanted the same things. Hopefully, they can continue to work together in the future.

Needing Routine Back

I WAS DELIGHTED to hear that I only had to drive to London instead of Toronto, where Dr. Ferguson came once a month to see some of his patients. We booked Jim's first after-surgery appointment for October 16. At this appointment, where only Jim was allowed in, he told the doctor about the unusual discomfort in the tibia bone of his leg. The doctor told him it was probably nerve pain, as the nerves were still healing. Jim also discussed his thought of returning to work in early November, which was fine with the doctor if Jim felt he could do it. Dr. Ferguson also informed Jim that he would need chest X-rays every three months to check for lung metastasis. He said this type of cancer moves from the leg to the lungs, so they have to be proactive to catch it.

When he returned home, I told him I wanted a weekend away with just him before he returned to work in a couple of weeks. I knew that he was so thankful for all that Premiere had done for him that he would want to make it up to them by giving it his all. So, after contemplating how far Jim could manage in the truck, we planned to go to Fergus for two days. A place not too far for Jim to drive to, we hoped. We had been there in passing a couple of years earlier and had promised each other we would go back to explore the beautiful town.

By this time, Jim would start his evenings in our bed but couldn't stay for a long period of time because of the discomfort he would get in his leg. So he would get up at night and sit in his comfy recliner in the next room to read, watch a movie, or look at the many photo albums I had put together of our family over the years. I could see he was very anxious about this night away. It would be challenging for him, but he was willing to try it, which I appreciated.

We got there in good time and walked around Fergus, enjoying being tourists, especially in the Dutch store! We went out for lunch and found a few local thrift stores, yet again showing our Dutch roots. While at a thrift store, people's cell phones were going off for a tornado warning for the evening. We were starting to second-guess our holiday. As we made our way to our hotel, we heard everyone talking about the tornado warnings. *Why do I feel I am not supposed to be here?* I thought. *I just wanted a nice vacation with my husband, just the two of us.*

Having settled our stuff in our hotel room, we went out for an enjoyable, elegant dinner. Later, back at the hotel, we had a good heart-to-heart talk about how life is different now, unlike it used to be. This was one of those talks where you don't say much because the words are too hard, but you both know. I remember wanting to find answers and solutions! I was frustrated. I could see in Jim's eyes that he felt almost defeated. He was hovering on that cliff. He kept saying, "I just have to get back to work. I have to do what I am good at doing. I need my routine back. Then it will be okay." My stomach was in knots as I snuggled up close to him. His arm pulled me closer as he kissed my forehead, and we tried to sleep. Later, in a half-dazed sleep, I sensed that Jim was uncomfortable. In the wee hours of the morning, he was up walking, trying to let me sleep while getting the knots out of his leg. Later he would come crawling back into bed, rearranging the extra pillows to get himself comfortable. By morning neither one of us had slept well. Maybe this vacation was not a good idea. We were both frustrated and not enjoying it anymore.

"I just want my La-Z-Boy," he said multiple times as the morning progressed, knowing that was where he could sleep best.

I argued, "I just wanted to look for a new mattress. You know, once you are back to work, you will be too tired to come to look at mattresses with me."

"I'm too tired now. I just need my chair." I knew I had pushed him too far. I could see the exhaustion on his face, and his limp was more pronounced.

"Okay, let's go home," I said, defeated.

"I'm sorry. I just can't do it anymore," he sincerely apologized.

"I know. I love you. Let's go find your chair," I said with a weak smile.

With November came the work routine that Jim craved. Even if it was only mornings to start with. He loved the fast pace of work, sitting behind the parts counter answering phones or helping walk-in customers who needed John Deere parts. He had missed all the banter at work, as they were like a second family. At one point, Jim and another gentleman with similar humour and wit to Jim's sat on each side of Melanie at the front counter selling parts. I remember coming in one day and Melanie said with mocked seriousness, "I am the rose between two thorns!" which brought on a round of laughter.

After a busy day of work in the morning, once everyone had lunch, he would head to his parents' house. He would sit with them, enjoying their company while eating lunch together. Sometimes he would have a short nap on their recliner before heading home. Other times he would choose just to come home and crash on his beloved chair for a long nap before picking some small job that needed to be done at home. He also contemplated what to do with Crispy now that the weather was getting colder. Let's just say Crispy was not an egg-laying chicken.

During this season, we had been staying home and watching church online. One Sunday Calvin asked if we could go back to in-person church. I told Jim that if my teenager asked to go to church, I would take him. Jim agreed but was unsure if it would be a good idea for him to go, so he chose to stay home. Walking into the church, sitting in the pew, and worshiping together was unbelievable. It felt something like coming home, but better. I tried to explain the feeling when I got home but couldn't. Jim cautiously joined us at church the following Sunday, wanting to have that amazing feeling too. Later, on the way home, he was in awe of how good it felt to be back in church, wishing we had done it sooner. From then on, Jim and I would be worshipping with others at both the morning and evening services. During this time worshipping in the church building, Jim and I felt ourselves getting closer to God, grounding us for the coming week.

When the new year began Jim was again working full time. As COVID was still a thing, we hoped our internet would keep up. Elly and Melissa worked on their university courses online upstairs. Downstairs, Calvin was doing online high school and I was homeschooling Joshua. Victoria was working with Youth Unlimited from home some days, while she searched to find a place of her own. The daily routine continued, and time passed as we kept busy at home, still unable to go out for extra activities.

Weekly date nights were a drive in Jim's pickup truck, going through a drive-thru, and working through our couple's devotional. These were treasured times for both of us. Not just a time to get out of the house but also a time to grow closer together and to God. It was also a time to discuss decisions we needed to make regarding the kids, with them out of earshot. It was a cherished time to create harmony in our marriage.

Hoping to continue the calm atmosphere upon returning home, we would try to get home after everyone was in bed. We should have known better. It didn't happen that way; their young bodies were more alive than our older ones. Upon entering the house, we still had to say, "Come on guys, off to bed!" It was not uncommon for Jim to sit in his chair and start flipping through his phone. Sometimes he would fall asleep there. As for myself, after getting ready for bed, I would read till I fell asleep. Often I would hear the girls whispering and giggling in the next room, where Jim had fallen asleep in his chair. The next thing I knew, they were carrying him into bed, or at least trying to. But as full-out laughter erupted, it was hard not to drop Dad, who was now wide-awake laughing. They always managed to get him in bed, under the covers, still fully clothed, sometimes even with his jacket on and crocs on his feet. Other nights, I don't know how or who would start it, but Jim and Melissa would be wrestling before bed. Many times, we would be going to bed, and Jim would sneak back out on tiptoe, turn off all the lights, and run back, trying to slam the door behind him. But Melissa would be thundering in after him, both of them laughing and wrestling. One night I found all my dining room chairs stacked in front of my bedroom door. Being the serious, not fun parent, I sternly insisted the chairs be returned immediately. I looked over to see two "children" pouting between giggles. How I wish I knew how to be a "fun" parent.

Wedding

FRIDAY, MAY 14, Jim left work late morning to see Dr. Ferguson for his routine chest X-ray. After the X-ray, Jim walked through the hospital to the waiting room to see the doctor. *Since this will be eight months, maybe they will let me come less often,* Jim thought hopefully, as he sat his tired body down in the waiting room. The line moved exceptionally slowly and Jim scrolled through his phone, sending the odd, funny YouTube video or photo to people at work or to me at home. Another gentleman who was waiting was getting agitated. He was talking about leaving since it was only a check-up. "But you know, this will be the one time that they find something. I told them, at work, I would be back," the gentleman stated in frustration. "This line is not moving!" Jim had the same thoughts but knew he had, and was thankful for, an understanding boss.

Finally getting an audience with the doctor, he was told the discomfort in his leg was most likely still nerve pain. The doctor said this was normal, as nerves take a long time to heal from surgery. In the meantime, he wrote a prescription to help with the pain. He also observed no sign of the tumours growing in his leg. Jim felt healthy otherwise, and neither had other concerns regarding his leg. Dr. Ferguson then proceeded to tell Jim that the X-rays showed a mass at the base of his left lung. An urgent CT scan would be ordered at Stratford Hospital—closer to us—within the next couple of weeks. Next month, he would have another appointment to discuss the results.

We could feel the rollercoaster ride starting up again. Lord, what is this ride going to look like? We asked others to join us as we prayed that the upcoming CT scan would show complete healing.

Sitting around the campfire one night around 9:00 pm after sending the kids to bed, Jim and I were enjoying one of the first campfires of the summer when his phone rang. It was Dr. Thornton, our family doctor.

"Sorry, I am calling so late, Jim."

"It's fine. Just enjoying a campfire in the backyard," he cheerfully replied.

"It's such nice weather for that lately," she responded, "Is Joanne with you, Jim?"

"Yes, I'm here too," I replied.

"Jim, I'm calling to talk to you about the CT scan if that is okay with you?" she questioned. "Or would you like to wait till your meeting with Dr. Ferguson?"

"No, I think I would like to know now, if that's okay?" he requested. I rummaged around in my pocket for a scrap piece of paper and pencil stub I had remembered fingering earlier. I prepared myself to take notes in the glow of the firelight. She revealed that they found a mass of 5.3 centimetres by 3.3 centimetres, roughly the size of an egg, in his lower left lung. With dismay, she told us of another smaller lymph node outside the lung that needed to be checked with an MRI. She would try to book that before Jim's next appointment on June 11 with Dr. Ferguson. The three of us agreed that if Jim had all the information he needed at this appointment, the doctor would be able to plan a quicker course of action. She anticipated it would probably include another surgery. I reached over to hold Jim's hand, squeezing it to let him know I was there for him. After he thanked her for calling us with this information, we said our goodbyes to Dr. Thornton.

Sitting quietly in the semi-darkness of the fire, holding hands, we both stared into the flames, trying to process the reality of possibly two tumours, or metastasis as they called them. Jim tugged my arm closer and I awkwardly moved my lawn chair through the grass closer to his. I just wanted to climb into his lap, hold him tight and cry. Oh Lord, help us. Tears rolled down my eyes as I turned to him, noticing the glistening in his eyes. He smiled weakly. Then together we prayed for strength in the coming days.

Think about it

This earthly world is full of hardships and sadness. Why are we surprised when hardship or sadness come to us? We can be in these hardships and trials with God, while looking at and rejoicing in the good, whether large or small. What are you finding hard to accept today? *"God is our refuge and strength, an ever-present help in trouble. Therefore we will not fear, though the earth give way and the mountains fall into the heart of the sea, though its*

waters roar and foam and the mountains quake with their surging"
(Psalm 46:1–3).

Tuesday, June 8. Jim went into Woodstock to get his first COVID shot with others from work. On the way, he heard on the radio that the government was increasing the permissible size of gatherings from ten people to fifty people. The ten-person limit had meant our large family couldn't participate in Christina and Cody's wedding set for this upcoming Saturday, June 12. But today that was all changing. Knowing it was short notice, Christina quickly asked all of hers and Cody's siblings to come. Most could make it, but sadly, a few had other engagements they couldn't break. Desiree went with me for the day on Thursday to help prepare Christina and Cody's backyard for their upcoming wedding reception, cleaning gardens and hanging flowers.

With the thoughts of the next day's wedding, Jim went to see the oncologist on Friday, June 11. I was able to listen in on the meeting via the phone which was an answer to prayer. Dr. Ferguson informed us that the tumour in Jim's lower left lung, the size of an egg, needed to come out, and he would be referring us to Dr. Fortin, a lung surgeon. We were happy to hear that the spot outside his lung, an enlarged lymph node, was unrelated to this cancer. He informed us that this is the best-case scenario, as it is only one mass, not many little ones, and is in the bottom of the lung, away from other important organs. It can be removed through surgery, with no radiation or chemo. Relief washed over me as I hung up the phone and waited for Jim to call me back when he returned to his truck. Then, Jim also pointed out that this operation would be in London, which was closer to home. We both felt better going to the wedding the next day with good—well, more desirable—news.

The long-awaited wedding day dawned with happiness in our hearts. The younger kids would drive the hour to church together, in time for the service. Jim and I went earlier to help Christina prepare—and, really, for moral support. Once everyone was ready, we all headed to the church. Upon arrival, Christina, her best friend Nicole, and Jim hid in the back room with our grandson Wesley, the ringbearer. Here Jim prayed over Christina and her marriage as tears filled all their eyes.

"Way to go, dad! Make my makeup run," Christina said mid-tears.

"You have time to pull yourself together. They can't start without us," Jim said through his mischievous smile. As they regained their composure, the groom moved from one foot to the other, waiting for his bride to come down the aisle.

Christina clung to her daddy as she walked down the aisle toward her soon-to-be husband, while the large sanctuary enveloped the small group. Being a relatively informal service, Jim and I had arranged with the minister that Jim would say a short speech and present a bible to the new couple. So partway through the service, the minister called Jim to the front as Christina and Cody's eyes shot up in surprise.

Jim arranged his papers on the podium, cleared his throat, and looked at Cody and Christina as he took a deep breath.

"Cody and Chrissy! Your big day has finally arrived. The day you can be husband and wife. Cody, today you take to be your wife, our little girl in pigtails!" The memory of Christina in pigtails running to greet him when he would come home from work was too much for Jim. Unfamiliar emotion took over as he looked down at the paper that swam before him. He pleadingly looked up at me sitting on the front pew. My heart broke for him as I pushed off the bench to help. *I'm the emotional one; how will I read his speech?* I thought, forging ahead to the podium to stand beside him. Taking Jim's left hand in mine, I looked up at him. He pushed his speech across the podium to me. Looking up at the bride and groom, who also had tears, I was thankful there were so few people present.

I began his speech again, "Cody, today you take to be your wife, our little girl in pigtails! When I—dad—cut the cord at her birth, he was showered with fluid, and she first became known as our squirt. As she became older, she would run to greet me at the door when I returned home from work as I called 'Lucy, I'm home'." Now it was my turn to cry.

Jim pulled the paper back in front of him, putting his arm around me and mine around him; he whispered, "I can do it now."

"At that point, she became, and always will be, my Lucy," he continued with a strong voice as he pressed on through his speech.

"Cody and Chrissy, we want you to build your marriage on faith. The faith that Christina was raised with. Faith that is centred on honouring God. Honouring God in your relationship with each other. Honouring God as you raise your family together. To do that, you need to be properly equipped. You need to always be looking for ways to strengthen your relationship with God who loves you, blesses you, and gives you his Grace. Some of the tools you need are prayer and worship. So, pray and worship together. And you need God's Word, so read it together. And so, in saying that, we want you to use this family Bible that this church is gifting you. And we as parents would like to present to you. A Bible that you can study together, and we pray will be a symbol of your faith as a family.

So, Cody and Chrissy, we present you with this Bible, and we pray for God's blessings on you as a family. We love you!" he finished as he handed them their very own bible.

After they were introduced as husband and wife, our small congregation filed out of the church and to the park for pictures and laughter. Then we went to Cody and Christina's for a backyard barbeque, where Jim stood flipping burgers and turning sausages. Here a few more friends and family joined us for a simple but enjoyable ending to a beautiful wedding day.

Covid Shot

TWO WEEKS LATER I drove to Jim's work to be with him while he had his phone appointment with the lung surgeon. As we sat together in my car, this delightful Dr. Fortin introduced herself to us, and from the get-go, we knew we would like her. (Jim also found out this was the same surgeon his boss had had, and he only spoke highly of her.) She told us there were three spots she could see on Jim's MRI that she would try to take out during surgery. Three? We were confused. We knew of one, the size of an egg, but two more? Over the phone, she tried to explain where they were and how the surgery would go. She informed us that her secretary would contact us soon, as they wanted to get Jim in as soon as possible.

Later that night at home, we worked on an update for our kids and prayer partners:

> This morning, June 24, Jim and Joanne had a call with the lung surgeon, Dr. Fortin, out of London. We were thrilled to hear that it would be a laparoscopic surgery, meaning they would only do a few small incisions and go in with a camera and some tools. This will mean minimal invasion and less recovery time. So, on July 8, Jim goes to Stratford hospital for a pulmonary function test to check out the health of his lungs. July 13 Jim, with Joanne!!, goes to London hospital for pre-op, sign paperwork, and physically meet with the surgeon. On Monday, July 19, Jim will have a 2-hour surgery to remove the tumour. Depending on how the surgery goes, he will be in the hospital for 1-4 days and be off work for 4-8 weeks. At this time, Joanne will not be allowed in the hospital on surgery day. She will only be able to talk to Jim via phone after surgery.

A week before his pre-op appointment, Jim started having chest pains. Out of curiosity, he started looking up some of the side effects of the COVID shot he had before Christina's wedding. After a lengthy chat with the family doctor, who had thoroughly researched it for her and her family, he was strongly advised to get the shot since he would be hospitalized due to his cancer. Jim in turn encouraged me to get my shot so I could be with him in the hospital whenever possible.

But this night, he was sitting in his reclining chair, trying to breathe through great pain. Always being a restless sleeper when Jim was not in bed with me, I finally got up to use the bathroom. Seeing he was awake in the moonlit room; I came to him and noticed the pain etched across his face. I asked if I needed to take him to the hospital.

"No, it's improving. I just need to sit still and rest. I'll be fine. I think it might just be myocarditis. It is a side effect for men my age. It will pass."

"But that was weeks ago that you had the shot."

"It says it can show up to three weeks afterward," he informed me while I calculated the weeks in my head, realizing he was in that time frame. After sitting with him for a bit, he sent me off to bed, where I lay staring at the ceiling, praying, and finally falling into another fitful sleep.

In the morning, he promised to text our family doctor to let her know what was happening. Once he was settled for the day at work, caught up on the morning activity, he made his way out to his truck for rest and privacy. He texted a short message to our family doctor, explaining the event from last night but that he was fine now, and he hit send. Before he was out of the truck, his phone began to ring. Looking down at the screen, he saw the family doctor's name appear and answered it.

"You get to the hospital *now!*" came the voice on the other end. After a brief discussion, Jim texted his boss to tell him he would probably not be in for the rest of the day, as he was heading to the hospital. And off he went, thinking this was a waste of time. He was feeling fine.

At the hospital, another doctor did multiple tests and said he couldn't find anything wrong with him. Jim suggested myocarditis from the COVID shot. The doctor huffed at him, saying the COVID shot doesn't do that. Needless to say, the doctor did a rapid ultrasound.

Jim said later, "He just waved it over me; there is no way he could have gotten any readings from that."

They kept telling him what it wasn't. Jim was frustrated because the excruciating pain was something; he felt it intensely. His texts to me showed his frustration very clearly. "What a waste of a day off work." "I should have never come to the hospital." He was upset, distraught. My worrying skills were fully activated while I prepared dinner for the family, and the kids sat oblivious in the next room. Was he falling into that pit of despair? The pit that has called some of my kids at times? It was a reality for me. I tried calling him to talk to him. He wouldn't answer, so I left a voicemail asking him to please talk to me.

"Jim, come home. You are scaring me. Where are you?" I wanted him to be okay. I wanted to hold him and tell him everything would be okay. Tears salted the meat I was stirring in the frying pan while I prayed from deep down. I tried calling again. It went directly to voicemail, so I knew he had turned his phone off. Now I was terrified. I turned the stove off and pushed the pan to the back of the stove. I went to my room and fell on my knees, praying, pleading with the Lord to keep Jim safe.

"Lord, please, *please* bring my husband home to me. Lord, I do not know where he is, but you do. Hold him, Lord. Keep him in your hands. Please, Lord, *please!*" I begged. Minutes trickled by, feeling like hours. I felt lost, not knowing what to do.

"I'm at the ball diamond," came the notification on my phone. I dashed to the bathroom, quickly splashing water on my face. I told the kids I was running out for a minute and would be right back. With only one thing on my mind, I ran to the car and sped the quarter mile down the road to the ball diamond while praying a prayer of thanksgiving that he was alive. As I pulled my car up beside his truck, many questions flew through my brain. Now what? What would I find? How would I approach him?

"Lord, give me the strength to be the wife he needs right now. Give me the words," I silently prayed as I walked to his driver's side door and slowly opened it. He lifted his head off his hands that gripped the top of the steering wheel and turned red eyes to me. We reached for each other, not saying a word. Sad and broken, we awkwardly held each other as I stood on the ground and he sat in the truck.

"Sorry, I just needed some time," he said after a while.

"I get it," I said, squeezing him one more time before letting go and making my way around the front of the truck to climb into the cab beside him.

"Will you miss me if I'm gone?" he asked seriously.

"Of course, I will miss you," shocked at his question. "You are kind of unforgettable," I snickered through tears. We talked for a while, then each of us took a deep breath. Agreeing it was time to return to being parents, we each drove home in our separate vehicles. As I made dinner, I thought about what Jim said, about me missing him. I needed to reassure him somehow. While Jim stayed close to me and me to him, for the rest of the evening, I started to come up with a plan.

Think about it.

Do you ever wonder why? Why does bad stuff happen to good people? Why do you or a loved one have to go through a hard time? God has a reason; we just have to trust him. He can see the whole picture; we just see a tiny sliver of that picture. *"His disciples asked him, "Rabbi, who sinned, this man or his parents, that he was born blind?' 'Neither this man nor his parents sinned,' said Jesus, 'but this happened so that the work of God might be displayed in his life'"* (John 9:2–3).

Over the next three days, every time I thought of something I would miss about him, I would jot it down. Some of them were:

- I will miss the shaving cream left on the bathroom counter in the mornings.
- I will miss the laundry beside the laundry basket instead of in the basket in our bedroom.
- I will miss you every time I snuggle one of our grandkids.
- I will miss your comment, "Looks good from here!" when I put wood in the woodstove.
- I will miss you when my washing machine breaks down *again*.
- I will miss you when I catch a mouse in the trap.
- I will miss your arms around me while I'm doing the dishes.
- I'll miss you teasing our kids.
- I'll miss your laughter that cheers any dreary day.

It went on and on. Three days later, I spent time rewriting my scribbles into a nice two-page letter. When finished, I folded it neatly and put it in a small plain envelope, hiding it in my purse. The next day, Saturday, we had made plans to go out on the motorcycle, just the two of us, before heading to visit Jim's friend Annette, now his aunt, and Uncle Rob at the Pinery after lunch. It was a beautiful day as we started our ride, zigzagging our way down the paved back roads to Grand Bend. Ending up by the park at the far end of the strip, we parked the motorcycle and started walking toward the beach. After a short walk, Jim saw a park bench and suggested we sit a while as he was tiring quickly these days.

After getting comfortable, I pulled the envelope out of my back pocket.

"What's this?" he asked me.

"Think of it as a little gift," I expressed tenderly.

Sending questioning glances my way, he worked the envelope open. He read through my list, then sat back against the bench, trying to let it sink in as he composed himself, not saying anything.

"The other day, you asked me if I would miss you if you were gone. I wanted you to know just some of the things I would miss. I'm sure there will be many more," I said as tears ran freely down my cheeks. He re-folded the letter, slipping it back into the envelope and then into the pocket over his heart. He stretched his arm over the back of the bench and around my shoulder.

"Thank you," he said, pulling me close. There we sat for a while, enjoying being peacefully close to each other without saying anything.

It was around this time that Jim declared he would write letters to each of his children. Starting with one and then another, he soon realized the magnitude of this project with ten children.

"Whose idea was it to have so many kids anyway?" he would say as the corners of his mouth moved up. "This is a lot of work." Then he would continue to write. It was not unusual for him to be interrupted whenever he sat on the porch to write, enjoying the breeze and his windchimes. There was always someone who needed to talk or hang out with dad, to tell him about their day or what was happening in their lives.

One day he announced, "I need to find a quiet place to write!"

"Good luck with that," I smiled.

"I'm going to the ball diamond," and off he went, paper, pen and envelopes in hand.

Think about it

I encourage you to write letters to the ones you love. Write about...

- Happy memories you had with them.
- The strengths that you see in them.
- Encouraging words for the days ahead.

- A bible verse they can cling to.
- Reassurances of love throughout.

"Above all, love each other deeply, because love covers over a multitude of sins" (1 Peter 4:8).

Meanwhile, Dr. Thornton had ordered a heart monitor for Jim to wear for forty-eight hours. She hoped the results would be in before our next appointment with Dr. Fortin. While he was wearing it, he thought it would be a good day to take the top of the old chimney down. While sweating up on the roof, as he lowered pail after pail of bricks down to the boys below to empty, the sticky tabs holding the probes on would let loose. This caused him to have to make the trip back down off the roof to find me, so I could help reattach the probes to his chest. Our neighbour Nick came by to see how it was going and offered his services. The next day, Nick was on the hot roof, and Jim was relaxing on the ground emptying the pail. The plan was for the older boys to redo that roof section in a few weeks. Jim's mom had already given him a stern talking to, saying that he was not allowed up there to help. When she saw that he wasn't heeding her words, she turned them to me, and I just shrugged helplessly.

"Do you think Dad would like it if we boys took him out for a camping or cottage weekend?" Nathan had asked earlier.

"I know he would love that since he is always trying to get you guys to go for a weekend camping trip," I replied. "Just remember it can't be too far as he can't sit in a vehicle that long." Nathan reached out to his brothers, who agreed to make it work. It was then decided that Nathan would reach out to friends from church whose cottage he had helped build. The cottage owners were happy to lend the boys the cottage, having followed our journey with our church family.

On July 9, 2021, Jim drove his truck with Nico and Joshua, loaded with food I had prepared for the weekend. They swung through Kitchener to pick up Nathan, who had finished working through the night, on their way to Cheer Lake. Derek picked up Calvin after finishing up early at work and headed up separately in the early afternoon.

Kayaking, canoeing, and swimming were only some of the highlights for the boys. Jim joined in some canoeing but spent a lot of time sitting on the shore, watching and laughing at the boys' antics. He did most of the cooking while the boys took turns helping. The main highlight for Jim was the ongoing card game of Wizard which caused much laughter. Upon returning home, Jim, smiling, spent many days replaying all the videos and looking through photos he had taken of the boys' adventures. It was clear to see that he had enjoyed this time immensely.

That following Tuesday, Jim and I met with Dr. Fortin at her clinic for Jim's pre-op appointment. She entered the room with a stack of paperwork in hand.

"What is the big idea going into the emergency department since our last chat, making me read all this paperwork?" she questioned with laughter in her voice. While she sat down in the chair to the left of us, she leafed through the stack of papers in her hands. She asked Jim to tell her what happened that brought him into the emergency room the week before. Attentively she listened to Jim, asking questions here and there. At one point, she noticed his crossed legs and told him not to cross them anymore. When asked why, she informed us that it could cause blood clots, which he didn't want.

Once she understood what was happening, she pulled out a drawing of a set of lungs from the stack of papers in her hands. With easy-to-understand terms, she explained to us while drawing on the diagram. In these details, we could see that the egg-sized metastasis was in the lower lobe of the left lung.

"It will be easy to remove since it is close to the outside," she confidently informed us. "There is another small one on the other side of the same lung here," she said as she drew another small circle to the right of the bigger circle, "which I also don't see as a problem." She explained that with laparoscopic surgery they go in and put a type of blanket around the metastasis. This blanket would contain the metastasis before they bring it out through the small incision they made for the tools.

"Now for the difficult one," she said, looking back down at the diagram while drawing a medium-sized circle by the heart. "This one appears to be in the fatty tissue around your heart. Due to your emergency room visit and what you told me, I feel I need more time to talk to the heart doctor for his opinion. I don't want to be all crazy and jump right in. I don't like surprises. I want to be prepared. But I want to be honest with you. This one is close to your aorta; waiting too long can make removing it more difficult. If it is okay with you, I would like to move the surgery date back one week," she expressed, waiting for our reply. We looked at each other and nodded our agreement while Jim stated that he just wanted it out.

Understanding Jim's eagerness, she continued by telling us it would be a three-hour surgery followed by a 2 to 3-day hospital stay before being able to go home. During our visit, as I watched her explain all this information and the risks involved, I was struck by the fact that she kept stopping to see if Jim understood. She waited for his response each time, looking intently at him, trying to read his body language. She didn't rush us or push us through. What doctor does that? You could see she cared.

Trying to keep our minds busy, we decided to keep our "camping reservation" at Hobo Hollow, a very private campground at Jim's cousin's farm. There was hydro, but all the water had to be brought in. Jim and I, and the two youngest boys and their friends would hang out here for the weekend.

The following week the lung surgeon called to say she talked to the heart doctor about Jim's tests. She confirmed the surgery would happen the next Monday. Jim was thankful, as he was getting more and more uncomfortable and sleeping was becoming more difficult.

Lung Surgery

IN THE EARLY hours of the day of the surgery, after a restless sleep, Jim and I began to get ready for the day. With butterflies in our stomachs, I finished dressing while Jim, already dressed, reached for the letters he had written for the kids. Pulling one out, he quietly walked around the bed to my side and slipped an envelope under my pillow.

"For you to read later," he said when he noticed I was watching him. "Can you give these other ones to the kids for me?" he self-consciously requested.

"You can give it to them when you see them next time," I reassured him.

"No, I want you to give it to them for me."

"You could mail them. I'll get some stamps," I said while going to the desk in our room to get the book of stamps I kept handy.

"No! I need you to give it to them," he stressed, "Promise me you will give them their letters."

"Fine. Because I love you, I'll make sure they all get them," I gave in as he pulled me into a hug. I pulled him tighter, not wanting to let go, both of us standing in each other's arms.

A little later, while sitting quietly in the passenger seat, my mind went back seventeen years to when Jim drove me to London for my surgery to remove a brain tumour. Remembering the need to find something to talk about, something funny, anything, I asked him if he felt the same as I had all those years ago. He confessed he did and then proceeded to tell me about some things I would need to know about the house.

"In January, you will have to check the wood stove chimneys. The living room chimney is very fragile. You will have to use the long flat screwdriver and be very careful. Don't take the cap off the top; leave it on," he started as I fished in my purse for a pen and a notepad. "The dining room one can twist off to clean and then just twist it back on."

"I'm not going up there," I declared. "I can do the living room one, but the dining room is way too high for my liking."

"Well, just ask the boys to help," he said with confidence.

"You need high-heat silicone to reseal the glass in the wood stove doors. Just make sure it's cool first and give it time to dry," he said. I could picture the many times he had done it in the past, feeling it was something I could do. "If the glass breaks, just go to Sam's Hardware for a new piece," which I already knew, having gotten the last piece there myself. I kept writing.

He went on to tell me about the snowblower, water softener, water filters, furnace and where to get wood, followed by who I was to call to get the septic cleaned and if I had a plumbing issue. I continued to jot down notes as he moved on to the vehicles. Once in a while I asked questions as he talked.

"Change the car oil and filter every five thousand kilometres and the truck every ten thousand kilometres. In the spring, do all the filters, cabin and engine air filters. The spark plugs were just done in the truck and must be done every couple of years."

"The snowblower switch needs to be fixed."

"So does the windshield in the truck," I reminded him.

"Yeah, that can be done by Apple Auto Glass," he noted. "Maybe you can ask your dad to touch up the rust spots on your car since he likes doing bodywork," he suggested.

"I'll ask him," I replied as we approached the hospital. Putting away the pen and notebook, we agreed he would pull up by the door, and I would switch to the driver's seat since I wouldn't be allowed to stay. Jim, not wanting to be caught twiddling his thumbs this time, grabbed the Reader's Digest he took from his mom and his phone, while I circled the car. Knowing neither of us wanted to let go; we gave each other a quick hug and went our separate ways. I climbed into the car, getting buckled in, while I watched him cross over to the hospital door and disappear.

As I pulled back into traffic, fresh tears slid down my cheeks. Would I see him again? "Lord, please send your angels to surround him. Please be with the doctors and nurses as they work on him today," I prayed as I headed home.

I made a short stop at home to pick up Jim's letters. Grabbing some stamps, I addressed and stamped Desiree and Christina's letters as they lived farther away. I put Joshua, Calvin, Melissa and Elly's letters on their beds. I would have to hand out the rest the next time I saw them. With that in mind, I went to Exeter to pick up my granddaughter Allie, then back to Fullarton to pick up my other granddaughter Chloe. These girls were a balm to my sad and hurting heart as they chirped excitedly from the back seat. Today was the first day of our church's Vacation Bible School (VBS). This event was run by my daughter Victoria with the help of Zoom. Fully equipped craft and activity supply bags were picked up beforehand that included a Zoom link to the program. We had delivered some of the bags to my daughter Desiree's family in Niagara, so her three kids could join in the fun too. The morning was full of children's laughter and giggles as they were unaware of the seriousness of their Papa's surgery.

After the morning program was over and the other kids had signed out, Victoria, Desiree and I stayed on Zoom to chat a little longer. Promising to let them know when I heard anything, I signed out to prepare lunch for the girls. Nervous, knowing the surgery would be about done, I jumped when the phone finally rang.

"The surgery went well. Jim is in the recovery room now. We had someone with paddles standing over him the whole time, but we are thankful we did not need them. The one by the lining of his heart was attached to his lung making us pretty confident that it is a metastasis and we were able to remove it with no issues. We removed the big metastasis but needed a larger incision than originally thought. It was more like a grapefruit than an egg. We also removed the small one in the bottom lobe, but we couldn't get to the one in his upper lobe," she informed me.

My mind was trying to concentrate, to comprehend. So much information at once. He is fine. It went well. Paddles? This sounds more serious than I had thought. Bigger hole? A grapefruit? That grew fast. Does that mean a longer healing time? He won't like that. One in the upper lobe? That can't be right. What one in the upper lobe? There were four? Oh no, we are not done yet. This was supposed to be the last. There is more. More? Oh, how do I tell Jim? More?

"Can I come in and see him?" I asked as the questions kept bouncing back and forth in my brain.

"Yes, the nurse will call you when he is in a room, and you may come in," she informed me.

Struggling with wanting to know or not, I gave in and asked, "There is another tumour in the top of his lung?"

"Well, there is a small spot, but we are not sure if it is a metastasis or if it is just something else. It is deeper than the others, making it harder to get at. It would be too invasive, so we left it and will watch to see if it is something," she explained. "The best explanation is to think of your lung like a chicken breast. The metastasis is deep in the breast. Finding and squeezing out a small one to two millimeter metastasis is really hard. It is better to wait and see if that is what it is. I'm sorry," she said genuinely.

"Thank you for all you have done today. We appreciate it," I said before texting Desiree and Victoria that surgery went well and I would see Dad this afternoon. Finishing up lunch, it took all my energy to follow Chloe and Allie's conversation, trying to stay upbeat for the girls.

Having received the call that Jim was in his room, I brought the girls home along with the letters for their dads and headed back to Victoria Hospital in London. I headed into the hospital with a duffle bag of his clothes, toiletries, and a few snacks, which had been stowed away in the car earlier that morning. After stopping to do the COVID screening at the door, I made my way to Jim's room, following the gentleman's directions.

Entering the room, I immediately saw things were not good. Jim's face showed pain. His brow was furrowed, his lips dry and tight, and his eyes were glassy. He held his hand out to me with a "help me, I need you" look. I dropped the bag at the end of the bed and went to him.

"I'm so glad you are here. I think I'm going to die. The pain," he said, putting his left hand on his chest over his heart. "I can't seem to get above it."

"Did you tell someone?" already knowing he would have.

"Yes. The nurse said the doctor is still on the floor and will come back before she leaves," he managed while trying to breathe through the pain. I went to put his bag out of the way. "Where are you going?"

"I'm not going anywhere. I am staying here with you. Just putting the bag away so no one trips over it," I reassured him.

While sitting on the chair beside him, I quietly told him about our morning adventures, trying to get his mind off the pain. Slowly he began to relax, even snickering a little when I told him the kids didn't recognize me in the pre-recorded science class. The only connection was from Chloe, who mentioned that the professor and Grandma had the same clock and chalkboard. We both wondered how long it would take them to figure out that crazy Professor Shaboom in the white lab coat and the crazy yellow wig was their grandma.

Standing, still holding his right hand, I gently rubbed his head with my left hand. He rested while I watched him breathe, looking him over closely. He had a small one-inch square bandage on the right side of his neck from where they put in a shunt. This was in case his heart quit during the surgery; they could inject him with meds to get his heart pumping again. A picture of them standing over him with paddles preparing for anything jumped into my mind. I tried not to think of that. I thanked God he was here; he was okay. Remembering the larger bandage to his left side just at the bottom of his ribs where the "grapefruit" came out, I pondered how long Jim would allow himself to heal. Just then Dr. Fortin came in with two resident doctors flanking her.

"So, I hear you are having some pain Mr. Schreuders," she inquired, waking Jim with a start. After her apology, Jim confirmed this, and she asked him to show her where it was. I saw him reach for the centre of his chest, where his heart was. "You should not have pain there. I do not know why you do," she pondered, thinking about it.

"It does seem to be getting a bit better since Joanne got here," he said, as I also noticed a more relaxed face looking at me. He was still uncomfortable but not in the same pain as when I first entered the room.

"Well, we will keep an eye on you." Taking a minute to think, she then added, "If it gets any worse, you let the nurses know, and we will see what we can do for you, okay?" Smiling at Jim's agreement, she asked if we had any other questions for her.

Pointing to the drainpipe—"more the thickness of a heater hose," Jim had pointed out earlier—he asked how long it had to stay in. This drain didn't have a small round vacuum on the end like the one he had with his leg surgery. This one was attached to a plastic box the size of a laptop but about two inches thick. He gave a sigh of relief when he heard it would be removed before he left the hospital.

My mind was still struggling. I wanted her to tell him about the tumour they left in there. I thought it would be better to get this over with now and better from the doctor than from me. With heaviness of heart, I broached the topic in my not-so-eloquent fashion, "Can you tell Jim what you told me on the phone?" When she looked at me bewildered, I continued, "About the top lobe?" Recollection dawning, she explained to Jim what she had told me earlier.

When she finished, she asked if we had any more questions. All of us were looking closely at Jim as he pondered this new information. Slowly he looked up at her, shaking his head no and said, "Thank you for coming back to talk with me."

Apologizing for the large incision, she added, "Sorry, I just couldn't seem to fit a grapefruit out of a pen-tip sized hole," bringing smiles to our faces. Telling him she would be back to check on him tomorrow, she, along with her sidekicks, turned to continue with her duties, leaving us feeling well cared for.

I stayed as late as I could, not wanting to leave his side. What if the pain was his heart? What if something happened if I left? Trying to overcome my fears and ease his, I finally made my way home in the dark with a promise to return.

Think about it

Any pain, discomfort, or grief at the deepest level, Jesus understands; he experienced it. Jesus died, for you and me, for the sins that we do every day; he hung on that cross. *"Surely he took up our infirmities and carried our sorrows, yet we considered him stricken by God, smitten by him, and afflicted. But he was pierced for our transgressions, he was crushed for our iniquities; the punishment that brought us peace was upon him, and by his wounds we are healed"* (Isaiah 53:4–5).

Hospital visiting hours were only in the afternoons. So I stayed busy doing VBS with the kids the following morning. After a Zoom time with cousins and a quick lunch, I returned the giggly girls to their respective houses.

Entering Jim's room on the second day, I found a much happier man. He informed me that he was feeling better, with only a lingering pain. They wanted him to keep moving to help keep blood clots from forming. So, we spent the day talking and walking the halls.

The next morning, while doing VBS activities, Jim got the "heater hose" out of his chest. When I arrived at the hospital that Wednesday afternoon, he was ready and eager to go home. Early that evening at home, one of the guys from work dropped off a fruit bouquet and a smiley face balloon bouquet for Jim to enjoy. While Jim sat down, trying to decipher all the names on the card, I tried to get the house back in order.

Finishing out the week of VBS, I tried not to overwhelm Jim. I don't know why I was so concerned, as he thrives on having people around. Their parents (my kids) and I instructed Chloe and Allie that there was no roughhousing with Papa. We had to be gentle with him. Coming into the house the next day, they didn't know what to expect; gingerly approaching Jim with concern on her face, Allie asked, "Are you okay, Papa?"

"I'll be fine, Allie," he said, reaching for a little hug. Smiling, she didn't disappoint him. He turned to Chloe, who had been hanging back.

"Do I get a Chloe hug, too?" he asked, creating a huge smile on her face as she melted into his embrace. I knew how these girls felt. I also wanted to give him a big old squeeze but was afraid I would hurt him.

"Just hug me. I'll let you know if I'm uncomfortable," he reassured me. He just needed to feel the love from those around him.

While Papa enjoyed his lawn chair on the front porch, reading and napping, we finished our week of VBS. It wasn't till the last day that my grandson Andrew, Desiree's oldest, asked if I was Professor Shaboom. With a smile, I neither agreed nor disagreed, leaving him guessing.

The Accident

ALMOST TWO WEEKS after his surgery, I drove Jim to the family doctor to have his stitches removed from the incision that held his drainpipe heater hose. The next day, marking two weeks since his surgery, he was allowed to drive himself around again. Unlike his last surgery, walking around was not an issue, so he informed me that he would visit his mom and dad and take... you guessed it, his motorcycle!

While he was gone, Josh and I sat on the couch watching a movie. I glanced at the clock at one point, thinking he was gone longer than usual. *Maybe he just stopped at work, catching up with everyone there*, I thought. Time went by, and my concern started to climb. Finally, he walked into the room behind us.

"There you are. I was starting to worry," I said, relieved. He sat down on a chair to our left, joining us in watching the last three minutes of the movie. I got up to manually turn it off when the show was finished. Turning around, I stood directly in line with where he was sitting. Glaring back at me was a big white bandage wrapped around his left forearm. My eyes flew to his face, where I saw a sheepish grin.

"What happened?" I interrogated as my heart beat faster and my stomach dropped.

"Nothing much," he said, much calmer than I felt. My heart was thumping so hard I thought it would move me across the floor like a pogo stick, but my feet wouldn't move. I just stood there trying to figure out what had happened.

"You know that traffic circle on the way home from Mom's where DS Equipment used to be?" I nodded my head, recalling the newer traffic circle.

"Well, a guy in a big pickup truck was not paying attention, just following the guy in front of him. I was already in the turn when I saw that he didn't see me. I went to hit the brakes, but the already-leaning motorcycle kept moving away. The guy in the truck saw me at the last minute. He slammed on his brakes as the motorbike skidded past in front of him to the other side of the road without me. Before I knew it, I had done a tuck and roll and was back on my feet." As an afterthought he added, "I maybe said a few bad words."

I stood there planted, staring at him. I was mad he was in an accident. Then, realizing it was not his fault, I was relieved he was okay. But then I kept bouncing back to anger, then to relief—so many conflicting emotions. Finally, my feet became unglued, and I went to hug him.

"Ohhhh, watch where you squeeze. I may have popped open where my stitches were yesterday," he said with a hint of a smile.

"What?" I quickly backed up to look at the blood on his white t-shirt that I didn't notice before.

"The paramedic says I should probably get stitches at the hospital. Can you just tape it up?"

"Are you serious?" I said in disbelief and nervousness.

"Yeah, just tape it together. I'm full of scars; what difference will one more make."

Noting that he was serious, I went for the first aid kit and did my best, patching him up. He agreed he would go to the hospital if it started to look bad or infected.

"How did you get home?"

"I drove the motorcycle," he stated matter-of-factly.

Backing up and looking into his face, I seriously asked, "You didn't lift it, did you? You just had lung surgery!"

"Well, I supervised as the three guys in the truck behind me helped pick it up," he said, not too convincingly. Or was I overthinking it all? "Yeah, I have to do some repairs to it now." After putting on another shirt and pants, he headed out to the garage, and I put his blood-stained shirt in to soak, my nerves still on edge.

As the week progressed, the road rash on his arm improved, but I was a little concerned about the popped stitches site. At our appointment with the cancer clinic later that week, I would get the doctor to look at it.

After getting his chest X-rays downstairs at Victoria Hospital in London, we made our way upstairs to check in with the receptionist. Here we were again directed to the large waiting room with lots of windows and people in groups of one or two social distancing on the distanced chairs. While waiting, we scrolled on our phones, shared things we found, and listened to other people's conversations. A little later, as we comfortably waited in the doctor's tiny office—with maybe more than a few butterflies in our tummies—we reviewed our few questions for her. One was the incision site he wanted me to tape up after his accident. Her lively chatter suddenly stopped inside the door as she noticed Jim's large road rash scab on his left arm.

"I didn't do that, did I?" she questioned, causing Jim and me to laugh.

"No, I had a little motorcycle accident earlier this week," he said with a twinkle in his eye.

Looking down at his file, she noted his surgery date, "You were out on your motorcycle that soon after surgery?" she questioned in shock.

"Well, you said I could drive after two weeks," he boldly stated.

"What happened?" she asked. Jim told her the story while she shook her head in disbelief. Putting her hands on her hips, she turned to me, and sighed in a motherly manner.

"I know, right? If cancer doesn't get him, that motorcycle will," I frustratedly added.

Turning back to Jim, she asked him how he was doing otherwise.

She questioned him, "How is your breathing? Any chest pains or coughing up blood?"

"I do not feel like I am short of breath at all, which surprises me, considering I am missing a chunk of a lung," he confessed. "My chest doesn't hurt, and the only time I coughed up blood was in the hospital." He told her he could ride the stationary bike for 5-10 minutes daily without shortness of breath.

She then went over the pathology report. Everything was good. All the margins and edges around the removed tumours were negative. Meaning they had good healthy tissue. We were shocked to learn that the grapefruit wedge also contained another tumour. So, in reality, they had removed four metastases—mets for short. We were thankful that one was not still in his body like the one that was still too small to deal with in the top left lobe.

She again apologized for the one that was left behind, but it was just too hard to get to at the time. She told us that according to the scan that was done today, it has not grown. They will keep an eye on it.

"Do you have any other questions for me?" she asked.

"Yes, can you look at this site that blew open when I went down with my motorcycle? My wife is worried," he said, pulling the side of his shirt up while I rolled my eyes at him. Smiling, she took a closer look before letting us know it was healing fine; she had no concerns. Again, she asked if we had questions while she calmly waited, looking at Jim intently. We reassured her we were good for now.

"If you think of anything, please feel free to call my office anytime. I will get back to you with an answer as soon as possible," she reassured us. Smiling and thanking her, we all left the tiny room to continue our day.

Jim's mom called us on our way home from the clinic, wanting to know how it went. We talked for a few minutes and then let her know we would be over tomorrow to visit. Knowing that his mom always had to comment on the motorcycle—she thought he should not drive one because it was too dangerous—we took the truck to visit. On previous occasions before the accident, she had tried to convince me to hide the key or take the battery out. After the accident, she noticed his scab and asked him what happened. He always artfully changed the topic so she wouldn't find out.

Fourteen years earlier, Dad had a stroke. He could no longer walk or talk, but he was usually able to communicate with us in some way. Then there was Mom; in true married-couple fashion, Mom knew what Dad wanted and needed. During one of our more recent visits, I was helping his mom upstairs while Jim sat with his dad downstairs. When we suddenly heard Dad getting all excited, Jim was laughing.

"What is going on down there now?" Mom asked, hearing Dad's commotion.

"Jim must have told him a joke because I can hear Jim laughing," I reassured her, as we continued with what we were doing.

Later, on the way home, Jim started giggling.

"What's so funny?" I asked.

"I told Dad about my accident with the bike," he snickered.

"Jim, you didn't! How is he supposed to communicate that to Mom?" I reprimanded him, "He has to hold that in?"

"I told him not to tell Mom," We both burst out laughing.

Trying to be serious, I said, "You should have left him with a dinky-car motorcycle and pickup so he could act it out for Mom."

"Naw, this is more fun," he declared.

Some weeks after Jim's birthday in August, our grandson Darius arrived in our kitchen with a shoebox-sized box full of holes. Nathan, Tim Horton's cup in hand, smiled as he instructed his son to give it to Papa.

"Here, Papa," he said in his cute two-year-old voice, clumsily dropping the box on the floor by Jim's feet. Getting down onto his knees, Darius tried to look into the holes.

Jim bent down, "What is it, Darius?" gently lifting the lid—inside peeped five baby chicks.

"They are layers, so they have a purpose," Nathan said, laughing. "Happy belated birthday!" Our other two-year-old grandson, Wesley, was visiting and came over to check out the commotion. The two boys sat there with their hands on their knees, crouched down, watching these little yellow puff balls.

"You boys going to help Papa put them in the chicken house?" Jim said after letting the boys hold them for a bit while he supervised. With quick agreement, they followed Papa, who carried the box outside to our big doghouse turned chicken house. Getting the chicks all settled in with fresh food and water; the boys again sat to watch them while chattering to each other and pointing to the little birds. This was the beginning of the tale of Papa's chickens, the comic relief that we all needed during the hard times that were to follow.

Back in the house, Nathan told Jim, "Sorry, Dad, I think I gave away your secret."

"What secret is that?"

"Well, I was visiting Opa and Oma after work this week. I may have mentioned your motorcycle accident," he smiled.

"Oh great. I guess it was bound to happen," he signed. "What did she say?"

"Well, it was quite funny. Opa got excited and kept pointing at Oma as if he knew. Oma asked him if he knew, and he nodded yes. Then he laughed while Oma got all worked up," Nathan laughed. Jim joined in the laughter while he explained that he had strictly told Opa not to tell Oma.

Up and Down, Repeat

OUR USUAL FAMILY group campsite was still closed at the Pinery, so back to Hobo Hollow we went, the whole family willing to give it a try. There was plenty of room for the kids to run, play, and yell as no one else was around. Usually a tent-camping family, Jim was happy to claim the only cabin with a real bed. Friday we arrived late in the morning to set up. This included making the two-week-old chicks comfortable in the screened-in gazebo. They couldn't be left at home for the neighbour to check on, or so he told me. Once the chicks were settled, Jim taught our youngest two boys (ages thirteen and fourteen) how to drive my standard car while I cringed at the difficult starts. The smiles on their faces—when they got the hang of it—were precious. It's a memory I'm sure will not soon be forgotten.

On Friday afternoon, I had arranged to pick up a bouncy castle from friends for the weekend, as there was no water nearby for the little ones to play in. Later that evening, Desiree's family came, and while the parents set up camp, Papa showed off his chicks. Our single daughters decided to sleep at home and return the next day. The older boys came out for the day on Saturday with their families. Jumping in the bouncy castle, catching bubbles from a bubble machine, checking out Papa's chicks, and chasing cousins around was great fun for the kids! Well, maybe for the kids at heart too. We all enjoyed hot dogs, burgers, and salads with many different pies that Desiree had made to celebrate Dad's love of pie.

As everyone was leaving, the discussion turned to whether we would be coming back here again next year or finding another group site. Jim standing next to me, listened quietly as the discussion continued. Most agreed that we needed to find somewhere with a beach close by.

"If I'm still here next year," Jim said quietly for only me to hear. Shock took hold of me. "No! Don't say that!" I wanted to yell at him. But deep down, I also knew that could be a possibility, no matter how much I didn't want to think about it. I knew this was his reality; he wouldn't live to be ninety like his grandfathers. I tried to think about having him for five more years. Ten more years? What would that look like? Surgery after surgery? Radiation? Would he be sick and weak for all those years, or would he be healthy and in remission? I felt confused. "Lord, you know what is best, what we need. Just stay close to us. Lord, give us strength to enjoy each day you bless us with," I silently prayed while reaching for Jim's hand and pulling him closer, hugging his arm to my chest. We said nothing more because there was nothing to say.

Desiree, her husband Joey, and their three kids were moving into a new house. Arriving the night before, we loaded our pickup truck and Derek's trailer with larger items from the house. I kept track of Jim, ensuring he didn't do too much lifting. His lung surgery had only been five weeks ago. When the truck and trailer were full, Jim drove the truck to my parents' house for the night, as they lived only ten minutes from the new house.

The next morning, Jim said he was not feeling well. He didn't think he would be much help. We brought our load over when the new house was unlocked at noon. Our two teenage boys helped unload while I started washing out the kitchen cupboards. Not his usual cheerful self, Jim leisurely supervised and then took himself on a tour of the new house.

"I think I need to go home really soon," he said quietly on his way back through the kitchen.

"Are you okay if I just finish wiping out this cupboard?" I asked, noting the strain on his face.

"Why don't you stay, and I will just take the boys home," he suggested. Looking at him, I knew I had to stay close by.

"Just let me finish this cupboard, and I will go with you, okay?" I stated, to which he didn't object. Finishing, I rounded up the boys, and we said our goodbyes amidst piled boxes and furniture everywhere. I could see Desiree felt a bit overwhelmed with three kids underfoot and people asking her where she wanted things. But she could see her dad was not feeling well. We had quick goodbye hugs, and we made our way home.

Jim started to improve as the night progressed, saying he didn't need a doctor. He would just sleep it off. By morning I could see he had improved to his old chipper self again.

"Since you are feeling better, what do you think if I went back to help Desiree?" I asked him.

"Fine with me. I am feeling much better. Why don't you stay and help her for a few days? I can stay here and supervise the boys," he said with mischief in his voice. Agreeing was easy. It wasn't often that I got to help my oldest daughter, having younger ones of my own still at home. Spending time with Desiree would be a treat for me. Quickly throwing some things in a duffle bag, I messaged my mom to see if I could spend a few nights there. With everything arranged, I left the house and walked into Desiree's new house two hours later. Seeing her jaw drop upon seeing me made it all worthwhile.

"Grandma's cleaning service at your service," I said with a smile. After a huge hug, we got to work. Joey, her husband, had to return to work, leaving Desiree and me to clean and sort the house. I enjoyed cleaning, but spending time with my grandkids and daughter I enjoyed more.

Meanwhile, Jim started working on his "Chicken Condo," as he called it. In reality it was the kids' clubhouse he had built with the older kids twenty-three years earlier. Never having been insulated, he was now cutting one piece of thick foam insulation at a time, ensuring that each piece fit snugly and tight between the studs.

The kids would laugh and say, "You never insulated it for us!"

To which Jim replied, "But these are my girls!"

"What are we?" his five daughters would declare with mocked shock.

"Ya, you're important too," he would wave his hand at them and laugh.

After the insulation was complete, he lowered the condo from its original height—six feet off the ground for head clearance—to four feet, so it was still off the ground, but he could get in and out easier. He then asked Nathan, one of our two carpenter sons, to build him a set of stairs to replace the ladder. Nathan obliged happily and worked on it one Saturday morning as his two kids and Papa supervised.

Jim went by himself to the heart specialist in early September. They did more in-depth studies of his heart and concluded it was fine. Jim then asked the specialist if it could have been from the COVID shot, but he would neither confirm nor deny this. The specialist went on to say that he saw no reason why Jim couldn't go for his second shot. So on his way home Jim stopped at the walk-in clinic in St. Marys and had his second shot, hoping he wouldn't have the same side effects as last time. He just wanted to keep his lungs as healthy as possible.

A week later we returned to Niagara for a weekend "camping" at my sister's ranch. My parents would be the only ones camping, as my brother and his family would go home to sleep and Jim and I would take the boys to sleep at my parents' place so Jim could have a bed. Arriving late in the afternoon, we visited while the barbeque was being prepared. Afterward, we had a big bonfire with almost all the younger nieces and nephews. Telling jokes and remembering camping trips of long ago, we all enjoyed our time catching up. As it became late, Jim quietly told me he needed to get to bed. So, collecting the boys, we headed to the truck with plans to see everyone bright and early in the morning.

Later that night, snuggled under the covers, I noticed Jim slipping out of bed. This was now a normal thing for us, him getting up to walk around to stretch muscles and to get comfortable as I rolled over and tried to get back to sleep. Almost an hour later, the call of nature also had me climbing out of bed. Climbing the stairs, I noticed Jim sitting very still in the recliner, staring straight ahead with his face tight.

"Are you okay?" I quietly asked as he blinked once and only slightly turned his head to me. I moved to my knees directly before him, placing my hands on his knees. I waited.

"My heart is racing. It feels like it is going to jump out of my chest. I don't feel good. I need to go home," he said fearfully.

"Maybe I should just take you to the hospital here," I suggested.

"No. If I need the hospital, I want to be close to home, to you and the kids. Please take me home," he pleaded.

"Let me go to the bathroom. Then I'll get the boys up, and we will pack the truck. You stay sitting. Relax," I reassured him.

"I'm sorry," he said quietly. "I know this was important to you."

"You are more important," I declared, kissing him while tears slid down my cheeks. This was our life now. The only constant was the unexpected.

I gently woke the boys, "I'm sorry, but you have to get up. Dad's not feeling well; we have to get him home."

"What time is it?" Calvin asked groggily, not wanting to get up.

"Around two o'clock in the morning," I answered, to which he groaned.

Joshua was up, quietly getting his stuff packed in his bag. "I'm sorry," I said as a new set of tears ran down my cheeks. "It's okay, Mom," he reassured me.

Once the boys and I had everything thrown in the truck, I returned for Jim and walked him slowly to the truck.

"You sure you don't want me to take you to the hospital?"

"No, I just want to go home," he repeated as I got him settled in the truck's passenger seat and headed for home.

Two hours later, we pulled into the driveway and he had noticeably improved. The boys went straight to bed after confirming that we would let them sleep in late. I texted the family to apologize—we wouldn't be joining the fun as we had gone home in the night. Once Jim was settled in bed, I climbed in next to him. Putting his arm around me, he pulled me close.

"I'm sorry I made you leave. I feel better now, but I did not know I would. I was scared it would just get worse and I would be too far from home. I am really sorry," he apologized again.

"It's okay, I understand. Let's just get some sleep now, okay?" I whispered, holding him tight and thanking God he was feeling better. We both relaxed for the first time that night, falling into a peaceful sleep.

Sugar and Cancer

WITH JIM BEING more tired, the thought of the metastasis in his upper lobe was heavy on our minds, but we didn't discuss it. Meanwhile, friends started sending us articles and links—"Sugar Causes Cancer!" Jim questioned multiple doctors and healthcare professionals about the relationship between food and cancer. Was sugar going to make it grow faster? All of them said that research shows that food and sugar do not play a factor in this type of cancer. Nevertheless, he had me book an online appointment with a dietician from the hospital. She talked about foods that would give him energy and what foods would make him tired. It seemed we were eating all the right things, except maybe the pie and some other baked goods. Should we take them off the list? I recalled previous years when I had tried to get us to eat healthier, even stopping the snacking after dinner. I was eager to see if it would be more successful this time. I thought we could encourage and support each other to eat better. But now, all of a sudden, like night and day, he could do it while I struggled.

A friend offered Jim a book which implied that he could get well with their ten-day plan. It came with a CD of music, another with scripture verses, and tear-away scripture memory cards. Inside, Jim read how healing was God's will. We had a problem with this book.

A few other chapters caught his attention, too, but probably not for the reason you are thinking. You see, Jim and I wholeheartedly believe that God has a reason for everything that happens. Theologically, we call this the "providence of God." Some times we might see the reason why things happen, but other times we may never see why. This is where *trust* (faith) really comes in. We trust that God, seeing the big picture, knows this is where we need to be right now. This is what we need to be going through. There is *hope* in this kind of trust.

Maybe God doesn't want to heal in this instance. Perhaps a better way to understand it is to trust that in God's big-picture plan healing might not be what is best. We have to trust Him. This book, and others like it, talk about things that block or prevent healing like sin, disobedience, unforgiveness and unbelief. For Jim and I this is bad theology. It's partially true; we are called to put those things to death. But we're fallen human beings, and no one is perfect. So, according to our understanding of this book, no one will ever be healed, because no one can live perfectly.

On the surface it sounds inspiring, but it's actually hopeless. If your loved one isn't granted healing, you're left thinking it's because you, or they, weren't good enough. You'll think, "I didn't think positively enough. I didn't believe it enough." It feels like it is all your fault. Where is the hope in that? The book has lots of good Bible verses and is well put together, but in the end, it's hopeless. Instead, believe God has a plan, and trust Him with whatever the outcome.

This way of thinking brought about much discussion with those who came to visit. The minister, and later different elders and friends, were all asked their views by Jim. These discussions strengthened his hope in the creator of the universe, who is here today and tomorrow, preparing the way for us. It made Jim, and me, as I listened to him, *hope filled*.

Think about it

When your loved ones "fall asleep," do you have the hope of seeing them again some day? Or will you grieve their loss with no hope? Hope gives energy; it keeps you going. Only you can secure that hope by having a personal relationship with Jesus. *"Brothers, we do not want you to be ignorant about those who fall asleep, or to grieve like the rest of men, who have no hope. We believe that Jesus died and rose again and so we believe that God will bring with Jesus those who have fallen asleep in him"* (1 Thessalonians 4:13–14).

To Have and to Hold

LATE SEPTEMBER 2021, as things were clamping down again due to COVID, we had a phone appointment with Dr. Fortin. She asked how Jim's breathing was and if he had chest pains or was coughing up blood. He told her he was fine and had resumed going back to work in the mornings.

Pleased with this report, she went on to talk about the metastasis that was still in his lung. We had learned that metastasis can only be found on an X-ray by comparing it to the last X-ray. By doing this, they not only found that the one in Jim's upper left lobe had grown by a millimetre or two, but so had the one in the upper right that they hadn't noticed before. She felt justified telling us these were not growing fast— we had time to figure out what to do. What bothered her most was the third one—yes, a third—in the right middle lobe.

"These lesions are still five to six millimetres and do not need to be treated immediately. However, the fact that two have grown and one is new is very suspicious for ongoing disease," she communicated. This new one was close enough to the outside of the lung for her to take out with surgery. But the other two smaller ones were really deep and taking them out would cause harm. She asked Jim's permission to consult with Dr. Lang (radiation doctor) and Dr. Logan (chemo doctor), who were more knowledgeable about this disease, to help make a plan. This is what we liked about this system. You had a team of doctors, some of whom we had never seen, all working for you. We hadn't yet met Dr. Logan, the chemo doctor. We had nothing against her, but we knew seeing her meant we were at the end of our rope. Leaving this phone appointment with the knowledge that they would do a follow-up scan in two to three months, we felt assured Jim's team of doctors were working together to make a good plan. But these tumours made us nervous.

"Is this what Dr. Ferguson meant when he said, 'At least it's not a whole bunch of little ones?'" Jim voiced the thoughts I had been thinking. "What is a whole bunch anyway?" he asked me, to which I could only shrug.

Jim and I began mulling over how we would celebrate our thirty-second anniversary. As October 7th was a weekday, we knew he wouldn't be taking off work. He was only working mornings, coming home after lunch. During the afternoons he usually had a nap and then would work on getting his energy and strength back, either on the relic of a stationary bike we had or on the elliptical machine our son Nicolas lent us. We agreed that after work and a nap, we would go out for a late lunch at the Cowbell Brewing Co. and then do something. What, we didn't know, but something. That's one thing Jim has taught me over the years. Let it go. Roll with it. Some days I still want to be in control, to plan. But I'm learning; deep breath and let it go.

On the morning of our anniversary, I received a phone call from Dr. Fortin. The team had agreed that radiation was the route to take for the three new metastases. I messaged Jim at work so he could inform his boss, and formulated another short email to send out.

That afternoon, he came in from work with a smile on his face and a bounce in his step. I could see he was looking forward to our date as much as I was.

"Ready to go?" he asked.

"Yes, but aren't you going to have a nap first?"

"I'm too excited to nap," he declared, sweeping me into his arms. "Come away with me, my love!" he whispered, looking deep into my eyes and making me light-headed with a passionate kiss.

"Ewww! Do you have to do that here?" Calvin said while dry heaving.

"Yeah. Really? Get a room," said Melissa. Jim smiled down at me and wiggled his eyebrows. I giggled as he found my hand and led me to the waiting truck.

As we drove toward Blythe, we commented on the beautiful fall colours.

"We should have gone for a drive north last weekend; the leaves will probably be done this weekend. They always finish up north before they do here," I said.

"Yeah. It's too bad. I like this time of year with all the colours." He reminisced with his own thoughts for a bit.

"So, what do you want to do after lunch?" he questioned.

"What about driving north and looking at the colours?" I proposed, thinking it would be relaxing enough for him, and we could stop and walk when he needed to stretch his leg.

"Really? I was thinking about this place up by Owen Sound. I remember going there a long time ago with the youth from church. Maybe we can find it back?"

Knowing I would surprise him with my spontaneity, I answered, "Sure, let's do it!" He smiled at me and readjusted his body in the seat behind the steering wheel as we pulled into the Cowbell parking lot. Even though it was a little cool, we agreed it was safer to sit out on the patio. I went into the building and asked for a table for two on the patio. Jim, having stayed outside, walked around the building, meeting the hostess and me as she showed me our table. Before heading for the long, colourful drive north, we enjoyed a late lunch and Jim's longed-for beer platter. Enjoying the sights and sharing our thoughts or enjoying periods of silence, the time ticked by.

"I think this is it," he announced as we pulled into a short driveway with a sign for Inglis Grist Mill. Pulling up to the booth, the cheerful young lady let us know that we were welcome to walk around, but the buildings were closing in five minutes. It was almost five o'clock. Where had the time gone? Easily finding a parking spot in the nearly empty parking lot, Jim confirmed this was the right place. We got out and walked to the top of a gorgeous waterfall. We took some selfies, laughing at how we were turning into our kids. Jim then suggested we walk down the trail.

"I'm sure this will bring us to the bottom of the falls. I remember being able to walk on the rocks down there," he recalled. I followed him down the well-worn trail. We zigzagged through boulders and hopped over crevices on an easy walking path, making our way gradually lower and lower. Then the path moved away from the falls, and he stopped, looking intently around. Like a hound dog, he returned to the falls muttering to himself.

"It is here somewhere. It has to be."

"What exactly are you looking for?" I asked him.

"There used to be a trail down this way somewhere. I remember it. It took you right down to the bottom."

"But the trail goes this way now," I urged to ears that were not hearing.

"Here, over here! I think this is it," he said with glee.

I looked down the hill, more of a mini cliff, really. "We can't climb down there! Yes, we could go down, but we would never get back up here again."

"Sure, we can! It's like steps." Then I noticed where he was looking. It was like steps between two boulders, steeper steps but very doable. Following him, we slowly took the steps while just fitting between the boulders.

"Are you going to be able to climb back up these?" I asked, thinking about how challenging regular stairs were for him.

"I was just thinking that too. But I think with the rocks on each side, I can use them to pull myself back up." Then he added as an afterthought, "or you will just have to pull me up."

"Depends on how nice you are to me. I know how you are with getting me in water."

"Yeah, remember when I accidentally tipped the canoe on our canoe trip with Joe and Cindy? You and all our stuff got soaking wet," he chuckled. "You were not happy with me."

Knowing he was following my thoughts, I stated, "We hadn't even pushed off-shore yet. I still can't believe you did that." I didn't find it funny at the time. But now I tried to hide the fact that, in retrospect, I could see the humour in the situation.

"You just sat there, in the front of the canoe, with water and fish swimming all around you," he laughed harder, turning to look at me. My laugh was short-lived as I lost my footing and let out a little scream, tumbling toward his arms as he caught me.

"Okay, enough talking. I have to concentrate," I said after he hugged me and gave me a quick kiss.

"Me too. This is more work than I thought," he confessed.

"You okay?"

"Yes, and we are almost there," he cheerfully announced.

We helped each other over the big rocks to the bottom of the falls. Once at the bottom, we found a large boulder to sit on in the middle of the waterway. Sitting peacefully, side by side, breathing in the fresh, crisp fall air, we watched the falls. The thundering waterfall ahead forced the water to run past us on both sides. There I sat, snuggled in Jim's arms as we marvelled at the creator who made all this beauty. Wanting to remember this day, we took some beautiful fall pictures and videos as the day grew later. With deep sighs, we agreed that we better return to the top before it got too dark.

With some difficulty and much concentration, Jim made it to the top with the help of the larger rocks along the way—and maybe a shove or two from me from behind. After taking a short rest along the trail, we casually strolled along the beaten path to the top. Once there, Jim wanted to try one of the other trails leading away from the falls.

"Are you sure you're okay?" I asked. His limp was getting more pronounced.

"Yes, this is good for me to work the muscles. Good workout for my lungs, too," he reassured me. I let him take the lead so I could keep pace with him. He reached back for my hand to pull me along beside him.

"You stay close to me, Mrs. Schreuders." Loved shone from his eyes.

"Gladly, Mr. Schreuders," I said, taking a quick step to catch up to him. At one point along the way, he stopped and looked around.

"What? What are you looking for?" I questioned, looking around to see what he might see. When I looked back at him, he was looking at me. He pulled me closer with a smirk on his face and a twinkle in his eye.

"Just making sure no one sees me kissing my lover. They might tell my wife." He grinned before giving me a kiss to remember. Holding him tight, we stood there for a few minutes till we became aware of another person on the trail. Blushing, I pulled back as he chuckled, and we kept walking.

"Remember that time your dad caught me kissing you?" he asked.

"How can I forget! I tried to pull away from you because I heard him coming down the stairs. But you just kept pulling me closer," I said, giggling at the memory.

"Boy was I embarrassed! I thought your dad would kick me out right then and there. But he didn't," he remembered. "Must have wanted to get rid of you really bad," he commented while ducking my swinging arm.

As dusk was upon us we made our way back to the truck, realizing we hadn't eaten dinner yet. Deciding on a light meal at Tim Hortons, we found our way into town. Enjoying each other's company, we talked about the past, present, and future. This continued a little as we made our way home, in more silence. Neither one of us wanted to go back, as the reality of our life was weighing heavy on our hearts.

On This Ride Together

A WEEK LATER, Jim, with no more discomfort in his leg or his lungs, headed back to London. His sore right hip made getting out of my low car difficult, so we started taking his pickup truck. Still unable to go into the hospital, I was left to write while waiting. Another CT scan had been ordered—as well as more tattoos—in preparation for his next round of radiation. They also needed him to do a breathing test. He was informed he would need to hold his breath while they did this round of radiation on his lungs. To think that they had to hit a five-millimetre spot deep in the lung with a radiation beam—little more than the width of a letter on this page! Of course, you didn't want the patient to breathe in and out.

Before he left, he was given a stack of paperwork. Tossing me the stack, he got himself comfortable in his place behind the driver's seat and told me they would let him know what the plan would be on Wednesday, when he returned for his first treatment. A mustard-coloured paper on the top of the stack showed the radiation start date and time: Wednesday, October 27. I started reading through the white pages about the radiation, much of the same information we received the last time he had radiation. Except for this time, the side effects were shocking. I read them out loud to Jim as he headed the truck back home.

"Coughing, difficulty breathing, shallow breathing and in extreme cases the feeling of suffocation… These symptoms may develop up to 3-6 months after radiation," I read with great concern.

"They just have to cover their butts, so they write everything that could happen. Don't worry about it," he tried to reassure me.

"Maybe so, but it is a little concerning. Sorry," I added, realizing I might be getting him worried and that I should keep my mouth shut. So instead, I reached down to my purse, took out paper and a pen, and started to formulate another email. After writing, asking for prayer warriors to help fight on our behalf so that Jim wouldn't suffer any of these side effects and that his hip pain would leave, I read it back to Jim. He again made rewording suggestions until we had it to his liking.

While working outside one afternoon, raking leaves and cleaning up the garden with Jim, Josh came running out the door.

"Telephone for you, mom. It's the school!" Josh yelled from the front door.

"Wonder what that's about?" I said, looking over at Jim. He shrugged as I entered the house to pick up the waiting receiver from the kitchen counter. Calvin's guidance counsellor's voice came through the line. Calvin was with her in her office on speaker-phone. He needed me to talk over some important things that were on his mind. The guidance counsellor could set up a special room for us to meet, as I would normally not be allowed into the school, but Calvin chose to talk in the car. After letting Jim know where I was going, I headed toward the school, arriving twenty minutes later. Pulling up to the front door, Calvin came out of the school and climbed in beside me. Turning off the car, I rotated in my seat in an attempt to face him. We talked about some things that were going on at school that the counsellor had mentioned. Waiting for him to get his thoughts, I sat quietly.

"Mom, is Dad going to die?" he blurted.

I took a long slow breath with a prayer in my heart for the right words. I reached for words he would be able to understand, but also needed to tell the truth.

"Yes, Calvin. Someday Dad is going to die. We do not know when. Maybe God will give him many more years, or maybe not. We don't know," I said gently.

As tears pooled in his eyes, he said, "I don't want Dad to die. It will hurt too much." I reached over and squeezed his hand that rested on his lap. "Remember Christina's friend who committed suicide?" he asked. I nodded, remembering how that death affected them. "Well, I still think of her lots, and it hurts. It hurts Mom." Tears welled in my eyes. "If Dad dies, I can't be here. It will hurt too much," he looked at me with pain in his glistening eyes.

In my head, my mother's heart pleaded with God, "Nooooo! Lord, give me the words to let him see this is not the answer."

"Calvin, you know that hurt you feel when you think of her?" He nodded as I saw him recalling the pain. "How do you think Mom and all your brothers and sisters would feel if we had to say goodbye to Dad *and* you? That would be a lot more hurt-ful. Calvin, we will all be hurting, but we will need each other more than ever. You will need to talk to us when it hurts before it hurts really bad. We will all understand your hurt because we will be missing Dad too. Promise me you will talk to us," I implored as my bottom lip quivered.

"Yes, Mom," he promised as I hugged him awkwardly. We wept together as I told him how much I loved him. When the tears subsided and we composed ourselves somewhat, Calvin boldly went back into the school, ready to finish the day. Hating to see my son crushed like that, I went home praying for him, and the other children who were on this rollercoaster ride with us.

Jim had vacation hours that he was told he had to use up before the end of the year, and decided to use them during his radiation schedule. As time grew closer, he started to get a sinus cold. Our concern was that they wouldn't be able to do the radiation. We knew it was a cold, but would they think it was COVID? This added some stress to the otherwise uneventful time. On the morning of his first treatment, Jim finally called the hospital and asked what the procedure was.

"Oh yes. You still come in. We do not stop for a cold or anything. Just make sure you have your mask on, maybe even wear a double one if you prefer," said the nurse confirming our arrival time. "We will see you soon, Jim." So off we went. Once again, I waited in the car.

Before I knew it, he was beside the car, hitting the window and scaring me half to death. Why do guys think that is so funny? He climbed in, still laughing, "You should have seen the look on your face!"

"Ha. Ha." I said in a serious tone, with my hand resting on my heart, trying to slow it down. After taking a few minutes to regain my composure, I asked, "So what did you find out?"

"Well, they can do all three at the same time, so we only have to come four more times."

"Oh good!"

"So, my next one is on Friday, then next Monday, Wednesday, and Friday. I just hope this cold goes away quickly. I feel that I need my strength, and this cold won't help those symptoms they are telling us about." He already looked tired.

That Monday we went to Dr. Lang's office in London for Jim's radiation review after his third treatment. The new treatments might have been going well, but Jim was starting to worry. Even though he knew she could do nothing about it, he shared with her his anxiety about the possibility of more metastases. She again mentioned that we should call the clinic if he started experiencing any side effects. She reassured us there was medication to help with most of these, but she didn't foresee him having any since the spots were so small. Jim agreed to book the next appointment for the radiation checkup in six weeks. From there, they would continue with CT scans of his thorax (chest) every three months, rotating between herself and Dr. Logan. We left feeling numb, with no real relief.

Friday morning brought us there once again for Jim's last treatment. When treatment was complete, only taking about fifteen minutes, we walked down the street in the frosty air to McDonald's for lunch. Taking it to go, we leisurely strolled side by side, heading back to the car to eat. About thirty minutes later, we agreed it was time to head back into the hospital to meet with Dr. Ferguson for a check-up of Jim's leg. I was allowed in for this appointment, finally meeting Jim's cancer doctor in person after more than seventeen months since his first appointment. After a short wait, Dr. Ferguson came through the door in a small whirlwind, talking before he fully entered the room. He asked Jim questions about his leg, noting that there didn't seem to be any recurring disease. Again, Jim mentioned the pain in his hip. And again, he was told it was a common side effect, still from surgery, and it would slowly go away over time. Picking up Jim's file, he told us that Jim would see Dr. Lang and Dr. Fortin for continued check-ups, and he would only be continuing Jim's care for his leg. He informed us that his receptionist would book us an appointment for six months from now. And he was gone.

"I get it now," I told Jim as we made our way back out of the hospital hand in hand.

"Get what?"

"Why I never got on the phone appointment when you first met him in Toronto." Jim turned to look at me with questioning eyes. "He means business. In and out, on to the next person," Jim smiled his agreement.

At the end of November, Jim was starting to feel pain in his lower left back. He was uncomfortable. Thinking it was his kidneys again, he started to up his fluid intake, hoping to wash the pain away. This discomfort didn't stop him from inviting Desiree and the kids, who were visiting from Niagara, to the local Tractor Parade. We also called up Derek and invited his family. All bundled up, we followed Derek's family to the dark back sideroad, a few concessions over. Here we all laughed at the Grinch and cheered for Santa as the tractor parade went by—yet another beautiful Christmas memory.

After the kids were in bed for the night, the sisters liked to hang out or play games together. One game that they sometimes chose was called "Write a line." Everyone gets a sheet of paper and writes a line. You hand the paper to the person on your right. They read the line and add another line folding the paper to hide the first line. The paper is again handed to the right; reading the last exposed line, you write another word or line, tucking under the one before. This continues until the paper has made a few rounds, depending on how many people are playing. When the original person gets their original paper, they unroll it and read to everyone what was written. Well, this night, Jim's paper made the room roll in laughter …

This year at Thanksgiving
Our little red hens
Were butchered.

This made Dad feel
Very very frustrated
Sexually speaking (please note this was Jim's addition)
Then again, maybe we
Can just forget all that and
Make popcorn with
Oil and heat
Give warmth
To the small innocent
Chickens with
Feet
Foot
Pain.

Another Wild Ride

MONDAY MORNING, JIM headed back to work full-time. With his vacation time used up, he had me book him an appointment with the family doctor as the kidney pain was not going away. Leaving work later that morning, he went to see what Dr. Thornton, our family doctor, could do for him. She didn't think it was his kidneys but needed to get a CT scan of his torso to be sure. He messaged me before returning to work and said she would get him a CT scan and message him as soon as she had it booked. She had written a prescription for pain medication that he would fill on his way back to work. He again mentioned how uncomfortable he was. Later that night, he got into his chair, and I got him a hot water bottle for his back. This helped relieve some of the pain.

Over the next few days, we noticed that the meds were not working. In the meantime, Dr. Thornton couldn't get him in for a CT scan. The best she could do was to add his lower back to the scan he already had scheduled for two weeks from now. She shared her frustration with us.

"You are home early," I said when Jim showed up in the kitchen at 4:30 Wednesday afternoon while I prepared dinner.

"I think you need to take me to emerg. I can't do this anymore. If this pain keeps up, I'll be dead by Friday," he lamented in anguish. I looked at the supper I was stirring on the stove and back at him, trying to figure out what to do next.

"Just let me finish this; it will be like five minutes. Then I will take you," I promised.

"Okay. I'm just going to sit here in my chair for a bit. Maybe it will improve so I can sit in the truck on the way to the hospital." As he made his way to the next room, bent in pain, I quickly finished what I was doing. I gave the girls instructions to finish preparing dinner, but Jim reassured me he would be fine until after we ate. After double-checking that he was sure, I finished making dinner. We ate while he stayed in his chair, not hungry due to the pain. He also mentioned that he would be ready if

72

he needed surgery. *He must be in a lot of pain*, I thought, after hearing him say those words nonchalantly.

The neighbours picked up Calvin for youth that night as I pulled out of the driveway with Jim beside me, both of us tense. Earlier, he had messaged our family doctor, who had instructed us to go to the St. Marys Hospital. Here we had an amazing on-call doctor who knew we were coming. He ordered chest X-rays and bloodwork. Pumping Jim with morphine helped the pain to subside as we waited for the X-ray results. Jim, more relaxed with the morphine in his body, could drift in and out of sleep until the doctor came with the results. He said he could see something but needed a clearer image, so he sent us to Stratford for that coveted CT scan.

Arriving in Stratford at midnight with my "happy" husband, amid the evening fog that had settled in, we slowly made our way down the halls to the quiet CT lab. I settled Jim in the lone chair while we waited at the door for the technologist, who never came. Jim's comment that he hoped the morphine would last long enough, made me anxious. Making sure he was okay, I walked as fast as I could back to the emergency department to let them know no one was coming. They called the lab and said she would be at the door where I left Jim. Hurrying back down the hall, I could hear Jim talking to someone as I approached.

"My wife is here. She just went back to emerg. She is coming."

"We can wait," she reassured him.

Rounding the corner, "I'm here!" I smiled as Jim made his way slowly through the double doors she had opened, relief registering on his face.

As I helped Jim prepare for the scan, the technician went into a room at the end of the short hall, flipping on a few light switches as she went. Getting everything ready, she returned shortly to claim Jim. I watched Jim follow her back through the doors she had just come from. Having a glimpse of the CT machine as the doors closed behind them, I listened to them talking and laughing as I pulled out my book to read in the empty room. Having trouble concentrating on the words as my eyes kept falling shut, I decided to lean back and get some rest. I could see this being a very long night.

Hearing the doors open a while later, I moved to put my book, which lay closed on my lap, back into my purse. I gathered Jim's clothes and stood as he made his way toward me with the technician close, watching his balance.

"Are you okay now?" She asked Jim. After he confirmed he would be fine, she turned her attention to include me.

"We will read these scans and return them to the St. Marys Hospital. They should have the results by the time you get there." We thanked her for her time as we prepared to leave.

Getting Jim back into the truck and buckling him in, I moved to the driver's side. Climbing behind the wheel and buckling myself in, I grabbed the wheel with both hands and took a deep, cleansing breath.

"Are you okay?" he asked.

"Yeah, I just need to wake up to concentrate on the road in this fog," I said.

"I can drive if you want me to," he said with a smile in his voice that I couldn't see clearly in the darkness around us. He knew I didn't like driving much, and it being late and foggy added to the stress I was already feeling.

"Not with that happy juice in your veins, you won't. Just keep talking to me so I stay awake, okay?" I asked.

"Sure," he agreed as we pulled out of the parking lot and made our way back to St. Marys Hospital through the thick fog, thankful that the roads were empty of other vehicles at this time of night. "Don't drive too slowly; I feel the morphine wearing off. I wonder if they will let me take some home. This is good stuff."

Smiling a greeting to our nurse in St. Marys, we found our way back into Jim's room; I tucked him under the single sheet. The nurse peeked in to make sure we were okay and said the doctor would be with us shortly.

"Well, we found out where all your pain is coming from," said the doctor as he walked into the room. "You have a build-up of fluid in your lower left lung. I just got off the phone with your thoracic team in London to consult with them. They would like you to go there and get it drained."

"To London, now?" Jim asked. By this time the morphine had definitely worn off. "That's another fifty minute drive. Can I get some more morphine first?"

"We could call an ambulance or, if you think you are all right going with your wife, we could give you more morphine for the trip," he suggested.

"My wife's driving has improved, so I think I'll go with her," he grinned.

"Well, thank you, Dear," I said, exasperated.

"Do you have extra morphine I can take home with me?" he questioned the doctor. "That's good stuff." Sadly, much to his disappointment, the answer was no. But he was willing to take what he could get as the nurse injected one last dose into the port in his arm before we returned to the quiet, foggy night.

London came with lights, noise and less fog as we pulled into the emergency parking lot. Making our way into the full emergency department around 4:00 in the morning, we stopped at the receptionist to let her know we were expected. I handed her the envelope with Jim's files which the doctor had sent with us. She slid it back and said to give it to the nurse when she called us. So there we sat, waiting. Finally, we were called and registered. Then Jim was taken to a back room; I was sent back into the emergency waiting room, and told I would be called back in a bit.

There I sat with Jim's paperwork in my hand, waiting. After about twenty minutes, I went to the reception, explaining that I was supposed to be called back and that I still had his paperwork. She said she would let them know and to please just be seated. Frustrated, I returned to my seat and waited. I picked up my book again to no avail. The room was bustling with people; how could I concentrate? I wanted to text people to pray, but who would be up in the wee hours of the morning? So, as I sat alone in a room full of people, I prayed. I prayed God would be with Jim as he waited inside, down at the end of the hall. Still waiting, I had a conversation with the nice young man beside me. Then I tried to figure out the stories of the others around me from the bits of conversations and the actions they shared. But for the most part, I sat, waiting, praying. I texted the girls at home so they would know what was happening when they awoke.

Around 8:30 am I had almost lost hope, when the double doors opened again. This time the nurse called for me. I jumped up, knocking over Jim's empty thermos cup. After fumbling with our coats, my purse, and the book while trying to sweep up the cup where it lay on the floor, I moved toward the door. She led me through a short maze amid construction, near the room where I had last seen Jim, before we came to an alcove where Jim lay behind a curtain.

"He is just coming to. You can sit here with him. The doctor should be here soon," she informed me as I unceremoniously dropped all the stuff on the chair that she had pointed out for me. Going straight to him with tears flowing, the long night was catching up to me; I looked at him peacefully sleeping. I reached for his strong hand that lay closest to me, gently squeezing it. As his eyelids fluttered, I noticed the freckles on his face for the first time in many years.

"Hey, handsome, how are you feeling now?" I whispered quietly as a smile turned up the corners of his dry full lips. He murmured something I couldn't make out.

"You just rest; I'm not going anywhere," I reassured him as I combed his thinning hair back from his face with my fingers. "I love you."

"Love you too." He forced the words past his lips with a thick tongue and his eyes closed again. I looked around him, finally taking note of our surroundings. There, on the floor beside me, was one of those "heater hose" boxes. It had red blood in it, measuring almost one and a half litres! More than what was in it after the two days following his lung surgery. A bit later, still groggy, the doctor asked Jim how he felt. Much better, he told the doctor. I hoped that was the truth and not more of the meds talking. The doctor explained that the tube had been inserted in the cavity between his lung and the lining of his lung. After a little more chatter, the doctor took his leave, telling us Jim would need to stay for a few days for observation.

"You should probably go home to the kids and let them know what is going on," he said with clearer speech now. "Are you going to be okay driving?" he asked as an afterthought.

"Oh, you would be amazed at what I can do on adrenaline," I tried to convince myself more than him. So, by around 9:00 am, I was on my way home, making plans for what I had to do at home before returning to Jim. Knowing that I needed to stay close to God in all this, I made sure I had a bunch of worship CDs in my car. While driving home, the old hymn "It is Well With My Soul" by Horatio P. Spafford, came on over the car speakers. It pulled me out of my random thoughts and sucked me in. The words washed over me as I reached over and cranked up the volume. With tears streaming down my cheeks, I felt the words deep down as I sang along.

Once it was finished, the peace that washed over me was overwhelming. I didn't want this feeling of peace to go away. So, I hit the replay button… twice. Then, taking a deep breath and praising God for watching over us no matter what happens, I continued driving with renewed strength.

After making a quick sandwich, I told Joshua to wake me up at noon and I laid down at 10:00 am for a nap. I forced my eyes to close, but my mind just kept spinning. I tried taking deep breaths and concentrating on relaxing each part of my body. It just was not working. So finally, I gave up trying to rest. I got up and prepared to talk to Jim's mom in person. After a big teenage sigh, Joshua agreed to come with me to make sure I stayed awake on the half-hour drive to Tavistock.

Amazed I made it without incident, we walked in, surprising his parents. Telling them the dreaded news was not easy as I relayed what had happened. Mom and I agreed that all that fluid was putting pressure on his lung and kidney. But I was thankful that I could assure them he was doing much better; he had texted me three of the most beautiful words: *Pain all gone.*

Each day I would visit him and he would say, "I just want to go home." Walking the halls was the only thing he could do, apart from surfing the web. Each day the doctor who had done the procedure—or perhaps it was his assistant—would come to check on him. Jim was frustrated because the man had an accent that he found difficult to understand, and he was not getting any answers. Each day he would ask the man or the nurses why he had blood in his lung. But he couldn't get a straight answer. He wished he could talk to Dr. Fortin, but she was on holiday. Disappointment reigned as he couldn't have the visitors he wanted; the ones who were important to him: his family. The new rule was that he could only have four visitors, all of whom must be vaccinated against COVID. He said he had the pastor and me on the list, so the kids would have to decide which other two would come to visit.

Taking his IV pole with him to hang his drain box on while not trying to get tangled in the "heater hose," we again headed to the hall. The hall in this part of the hospital had a "hill" up to the building it was attached to. It helped him practice working out, as it took strength even to climb this grade. On one of those first trips up, Jim mentioned another hill he would climb with the kids at the cottage in Grand Bend. The one where he and the kids would board the fat-tired wagon and ride down the steep street. One of his "Best Dad Ever" moves in the older kids' memories. Finally, he couldn't pass up the opportunity. He climbed on that wheelie pole and tried to ride it down the hall grade.

"Jim, you shouldn't be doing that!" I whispered in shock.

"Come on, everyone has to have a little fun once in a while," he smirked. From the bottom of the grade, behind the nurses' station, we heard, "Mr. Schreuders, I see you!" The attempt at a stern reprimand came from a nurse we couldn't see.

"You see n-o-t-h-i-n-g. I'm just trying to have some fun here," Jim said, removing his feet from the wheelie pole that had been pathetically inching its way down the hill under his weight.

On another afternoon, they allowed us to walk around the hospital, and we investigated the route to and from the cafeteria. Later that night, when I went to leave, my parking pass wouldn't work. When I pulled up to the booth, the parking attendant informed me through the closed window that her shift was over; she wouldn't help me. I backed up into a parking spot, I was stuck in the parking lot. I sat there thinking of what to do. I felt lost and alone as the cold rain and wind picked up around my parked car in the nearly empty lot. Finally, I realized the only option I had to get out of the lot was to pay with a credit card—Jim's credit card. I called Jim in the hospital, asking if he could meet me at the entrance near the pedestrian bridge we had come to earlier.

"Well, this would not be such a problem if you weren't so against credit cards," he rubbed in.

"Fine, I will consider it. Can you just meet me there so I can pay for parking at the bottom of the ramp and bring your card back?" I pleaded with him. I parked closer to the ramp and made my way through the cold pelting rain toward the tunnel. I saw him coming slowly down the hall with his wallet in one hand and IV pole in the other. On the way he made a comment to the COVID police that I didn't hear. Judging from their smiles, I probably didn't want to know. So I said nothing when I met him at his end of the tunnel. Taking the card, I ran back down the ramp and paid for parking at the kiosk machine. Grabbing the ticket, I returned to Jim and gave him a kiss while handing him his card. I heard him laugh as he watched me leave before heading back to his room.

On Monday, the fourth day of his stay, he sent a text in the morning asking me to bring the truck; they were going to remove the chest tube. I could hear the joy in his words. I arrived earlier than I had on previous days. Jim had another CT scan to ensure everything looked good. As we waited for the okay, Jim, dressed in his own clothing, was more than ready to leave. When the nurse finally arrived at about 4:00 pm with his discharge papers, he said, "We're outta here!" as he jerked his thumb over his right shoulder.

God's Hands and Feet

MEANWHILE, MORE PEOPLE were asking about Jim and being added to our prayer list. We were getting cards in the mail and emails from people saying they were praying for us. We got one card from a mega church near Toronto; we knew this because Jim googled it. The pastors and a prayer team of the church signed it. We had no idea how people there would know us. We asked everyone we could think of if they knew anyone from this congregation. No one knew. Would it stay a mystery? It baffled us. Until one day, when my mom mentioned that my uncle and aunt, whom I rarely see, had said to tell us they were praying for us. Jim grabbed the card off the shelf among so many others and showed it to her.

"Yes, that's their church," she confirmed. "Sorry, he told me a while ago. I just forgot. That was nice of them to send a card."

"Do you know how many sleepless nights I have been trying to figure this mystery out for?" he said with an exasperated sigh.

"Sorry," my mom said with a laugh.

Another day, there was a knock on the door. I opened it to find an older gentleman from our church standing nervously with an envelope in his hands.

"I just came for a minute," he said, stepping in to allow me to close the door, keeping the cool air outside. "I heard Jim is not working much, and I wanted to help. I'm too old to be much help physically, but I still wanted to help," he said, handing me the envelope he was fiddling with. "I would like to keep this between us?" he asked nervously. I understood the Christian mindset of giving in secret. I thanked him from my heart, and he quickly took his leave.

With the envelope in hand, I approached Jim as he sat in his reclining chair. I handed him the envelope. "What is this?" he asked, opening the envelope and looking inside. I explained to him the unexpected visitor as Jim pulled out $1000. Both of us were speechless. This was not the only time God had blessed us through other people. The school also sent grocery gift cards home with Calvin one day. We had another couple give us $1000 in gas gift cards. At church, I would find envelopes in our mail slot with gift cards and no names attached. We were thankful to those who allowed themselves to be God's hands and feet. People were so generous. This generosity released us to concentrate on Jim's health instead of where our next meal would come from or how we would make it to our next appointment. God was good; there was no denying that.

Think about it

God created us to help each other. Help comes in many forms:

- Gas cards for the trips back and forth to the hospital.
- Restaurant cards for days travelling to or from the hospital.
- Parking pass for the hospital.
- Grocery cards to help with the reduced income.
- Gift basket to the hospital with healthy snacks and maybe a book or game to pass the time.
- Meals (fresh or frozen) for times when we don't have time to cook or don't feel like cooking.
- Baking for when company comes to visit.
- Spending time with the kids and giving them something fun to do.
- General house cleaning and maintenance.
- Mow lawns, gardening or snow removal.
- Walmart cards for clothing and other household items.
- Canadian Tire cards for household items—we used ours for humidifiers to moisten Jim's lungs.
- Cash can help in an abundance of ways.

Accept help. Don't be proud. By accepting help from others, you are blessing them as much as they are blessing you. *"Command them to do good, to be rich in good deeds, and to be generous and willing to share"* (1 Timothy 6:18).

Looking better and getting back to his old self again, Jim started puttering around the house, doing small jobs and exercising on the equipment. But the nights were still hard. He was getting up in the night and going to his chair where he would read, watch a movie on his phone or look through the many photo albums I had made over the years. I would feel—rather than hear—him leave the bed as a gust of cold air would come in between the sheets. I never did sleep well without him in bed with me. He was like my security blanket. I would be semi-conscious, listening for him in the next room, trying to hear his breathing. I would chase away thoughts of finding him in the chair, but with Jesus. I would stop by to check on him when I got up to go to the bathroom. Sometimes we would have a little chat. Other times I would tuck a blanket around him and kiss him before going back to bed, where I would attempt to sleep alone.

Wednesday morning, I woke up declaring I had had enough. I didn't care how much it was going to cost. I was going to get us an adjustable bed so we could sleep together again. Always listening for him at night when he lay on his chair in the next room didn't help either of us get a full night's sleep. I knew that life wouldn't improve in this area. I needed him close so I could, I hoped, sleep again.

So that night, after dropping Calvin off at youth group, I went to some stores in Stratford to look at beds and get some ideas. I was shocked to see the cost of these beds! Maybe I did care how much they cost. How could we ever afford it? As I drove back to the church fifteen minutes early, I sat back with a huge sigh.

"Lord, I don't know what to do. I just want to be with the man you gave me," I said with a heavy heart, aloud in the quiet car. I reached over and picked up my phone, noticing a missed call from a gentleman in our church. Thinking I had some time before Calvin came out, I hit redial.

"Hello?"

"Hello. This is Joanne. You called?"

"Yes. Yes, I did. I was calling to see how Jim was doing. We heard in church on Sunday that he was back in the hospital?"

"Yes, he came back home Monday. But he is still not sleeping well at night. He keeps going to his recliner and finishes sleeping there at night. I was just now looking at ultramatic beds so he can stay in bed."

"You get one. I'll pay for it," he said without missing a beat.

"Pardon?" I asked, thinking I didn't hear him correctly.

"You guys find a bed you like, and I'm paying for it," he stated clearly.

"They are very expensive. Do you have any idea how much they cost? You can't do that!" I said in shock.

"Joanne, God has blessed me, and I want to bless you by buying this bed."

81

"O-kay?" I said hesitantly.

"I am serious. You talk to Jim and find a bed. I will be calling you back to make sure you pick one you like."

What was I to say?

"Thank you," I said with tears glistening in the headlights as parents arrived to pick up their youth.

"And Joanne, I don't want you to tell anyone I am doing this, okay."

"Yes, I totally understand," I said before hanging up. I remembered what Jesus says in Matthew 6:3, *"But when you give to the needy, do not let your left hand know what your right hand is doing."*

Needless to say, I was a little distracted on the way home. I wanted to explode with this new information. But I was able to keep it inside until we were alone later that night. Jim was also shocked but excited about the possibility of sharing a bed for the whole night again. Snuggling up close, we did our evening devotions, followed by a prayer of thanksgiving for all who were helping us through this hard time, ending with those whom we knew needed prayer also. I drifted off to sleep after yet another exhausting day, knowing that soon Jim would be back up in his chair to finish the night.

Getting Answers

THE NEXT DAY Jim declared that he was going back to work. I would have to trust him on this. I thought a half day would probably be doable, considering all he was doing at home. This would also have him home in time for his phone meeting with Dr. Lang. He packed a lunch and I saw him off at the door.

Christina came from Mount Forest later that morning to do some Scentsy deliveries in the area and to check on her dad.

"Well, he should be home shortly after lunch," I informed her. But as time passed and he didn't come home, I started to worry. Finally giving in, trying not to be controlling, I texted.

"So, when do you think you will be home?"

"6:00," came the reply. Was he going to stay a full day?

"I thought you were only working the morning? And what about the appointment with Dr. Lang?" I texted back in frustration.

"Nope. Busy. I'll take the meeting from here."

Throwing my hands up in the air, "Stubborn man!" I huffed in annoyance.

Later that day, after a full day at work, he confided that he had probably overdone it. Before Christina and her son Wesley made their way home after a quick dinner, Jim made himself comfortable in his chair again. He knew something was not right as he told me about his meeting with Dr. Lang. She confirmed that the pain was probably the fluid build-up. She explained that the fluid didn't have cancer in it; they were not sure where it came from exactly. She ordered another PET scan to be done in the upcoming weeks. Then they would see where they were with the disease. Leaning back in his chair, Jim decided that he needed to stay home tomorrow. He was kicking himself for sticking it out the full day.

By the next morning, Jim was even more uncomfortable. Taking Dr. Lang's advice, he called the clinic and talked to the doctor on call. Scared to let it get as bad as the last time he was in the hospital, he explained that it felt like the fluid was building up again inside his lung. We followed this doctor's directions and headed to St. Marys Hospital for a chest X-ray. Later that afternoon he called back to tell us that nothing was really different from his last one. He advised Jim to take his pain medication and follow up with Dr. Fortin next week. If symptoms got any worse, he was to go back to the emergency department.

In the meantime, we had arranged for a small Christmas party with Jim's family, since his sister Julia and her husband Henk were back from Saskatchewan for a bit. I was on edge seeing his discomfort and wondering if it would be better if we just stayed home, close to his recliner. He himself seemed to be teetering about whether or not to go, so I left it up to him. In the end, we took our potluck dish and headed to his parents in Tavistock to have dinner with his siblings and their significant others. His younger sister, Mary, and brother Jonathan had the four youngest grandchildren, who were also attending. Children always made for an entertaining dinner. Jim's older sister, Julia, and I were thankful we were through that stage. While there, Jim put on a good face, joking and teasing. I sat back, watching them banter about who was Mom's favourite, something that always happened when these siblings got together. They would each explain what they had done, exclaiming that this made them her favourite.

After dinner, Jim's sister-in-law Rio took some pictures of the siblings with Mom and Dad. They hadn't done this in many years and the picture would be a treasure. Everyone was smiling and laughing. It was a good picture, capturing everyone's personalities, a treasure for years to come.

By Monday, we were back at St. Marys for bloodwork and X-rays, and again, they sent us to London to be cared for by Jim's team. Jim just wanted them to put that tube back in and drain the fluid so he could be comfortable again; that's all he wanted. After a long, uncomfortable wait in the waiting room, they called Jim to the back, where they got him settled in a bed. Once he was in his beautiful gown and under the thin sheet, they called me to join him in the big room with only curtains separating the many patients. I felt privileged, as I was one of only a few being allowed with their loved ones. We couldn't help but listen to a confused senior as she repeatedly called out, "They are taking my money! Don't let them have my money!" It was not a quiet, peaceful place, with the murmurings of other patients, along with the voices of nurses and doctors that came and went.

They seemed to keep changing their mind about what they wanted to do for Jim. Finally, after many hours, they decided to do nothing. Jim would be brought up to a room to be monitored for a while. How long? We didn't know; they didn't seem to either. While he waited in the busy, noisy room, it was decided I would go home to be with the kids and get some chores done around the house. He would call me when I should come back. Again, on my way home, I struggled with how to split my time between Jim and the kids. I hadn't even talked to the kids much about how they were all dealing with Dad's situation. I made it my goal that night to sit and listen to where they were at. Even if it was just important-to-them stuff, I was going to be there.

Later that day, Jim texted me to say that he was waiting on more tests. "Just stay home tonight with the kids... I'm fine here... I really don't want to be here... They have me in a closet. At least it feels that way; the room is so small... I'd rather be there with you guys... I hope they let me go home tomorrow." My heart was breaking for him. "Lord, please let this be resolved and let him come home. He just wants to come home. Please, Lord!" I prayed over and over that night. At the same time, I began feeling a bit rejuvenated as I tidied up, getting the laundry folded and dishes washed. The kids were a big help, but it was not my way of doing things. (I had to learn to let it go.) Yes, the laundry was all washed. I fold clothes right away, but they don't. I tidy the rooms every night, but they don't see the mess. I wash the dishes after every meal, but they don't. It was just relaxing for me to putter with the everyday mindless chores, and get my house back the way it should be... for me.

Jim called me on my cell the next morning, "Are you on your way? The doctor wanted to talk to me, and I asked him to wait until you got here."

"I'm on my way!" I said. I had pulled over to the side of the road to answer his call. "Just outside of St. Marys by the cement plant."

"Okay great. See you soon, honey."

"Be there in a bit. Love you. Bye."

When I arrived, the nurse directed me to a small, short back hall where there was a supply closet on the left. Jim's voice came from the small room on the right, about the same size as the supply closet but with a window at the end. When I entered the room, Nathan was sitting on the bed talking to Jim, who sat in a chair by the one window.

"There you are," Jim said to me. "What took you so long?"

"Well, there is a thing called traffic! Not to mention the construction they are doing right here by the stop light." Moving to sit beside Nathan, I said with a smile, "They let you in, did they, Nate?"

"Yep." He explained he got off early from work, not far from the hospital and thought he would check on Dad. We had a short visit while we waited for the doctor's return. A little later, the doctor peeked his head in to see if I had arrived.

"She's here. We can talk now if it works for you," Jim informed him. Nathan got up to leave to give us space. Jim and I both asked if he would stay. We both thought it better to have another set of ears to hear what the doctor had to say. This way, if the other kids wanted to know anything, they could get his opinion too.

Nathan sat back on the bed beside me as the doctor left to get another chair. Returning with a chair in hand, he closed the door behind himself. After quick introductions, we discussed the four-people visitation policy and how hard that was with ten kids. Jim had the minister and me on the list but told the kids they had to figure out who was taking the last two spots.

"Do you let in support chickens?" I asked as Jim and Nathan laughed while the doctor sat confused.

"You are a chicken farmer?" the doctor asked Jim.

"No, well, sort of," he said, confusing the doctor more.

"I gave Dad five laying hens. He takes them very seriously," Nathan laughed in reply.

The doctor's lips curled into a smile. "Okay then!" he said and redirected the conversation. He reviewed all that Jim had been through with his cancer. Jim again mentioned that no one would tell him why there was so much blood in his lung.

"The scans all show that you do not have fluid buildup in your lung now. You might have a bit that has been absorbed into the tissue in the lung, and there is not much we can do about that. But we see no signs that we need to put another tube in right now, which is good," he informed us.

"Then why am I so uncomfortable there?" Jim questioned.

"The team has looked at your scans. We compared the ones from this morning to those ones you had done when you were here last week. It shows that the mets in your lung are growing faster, and there are more of them. They are out of control. I am sorry, Mr. Schreuders. At this point, the only thing we can do is keep you as comfortable as possible." He sat quietly while we let this sink in.

I stared at the doctor, dumbfounded, trying to wrap my head around what he had just said. Then I looked over at Jim, who was sitting quietly looking at the ground, thinking, processing. His eyes slowly found mine across the room, and my heart twisted at the helpless look I saw in them. I wanted to go to him, hold him, but I was numb. I couldn't think or speak. I followed his gaze as he turned to Nathan. He also was speechless as he watched his dad's face.

Jim turned back to the doctor, "So now what? Can we do surgery and just cut them out?"

"I do not see that as an option as that would be too big of a surgery. But you can talk to Dr. Fortin at your next appointment on Friday. Jim, you have to make some decisions. They do not need to be made right now unless you already know. But how do you picture the end of life?"

"I want to be at home with my family. Definitely not in the hospital."

"Okay, and if there is an emergency, do you want them to do everything in their power to keep you alive."

"Well, yes. I don't want them to give up on me."

"Okay, I want you to think about this some more. If you change your mind at any time, you need to tell your family and the doctor so it can go on your record. There are options you have now. One is just not to do anything and let it take its course, and we keep you as comfortable as possible. Second, we can get you in to talk to Dr. Logan about drug therapy. Or thirdly, we can get you to talk with Dr. Lang about more radiation. This option usually stops the bleeding of the mets in your lung. Sometimes it also slows the growth and might even shrink them for a little bit." The doctor seemed to ramble on and I felt like Charlie Brown listening to his teacher.

"I'm not sure. I want to keep all my options open, but I think I'm leaning toward radiation…. I think," Jim said hesitantly.

"I'm glad you are thinking about it. If we did radiation, we would like to get you in for radiation assessment as soon as possible. While you wait to talk to the doctors, can we start on a radiation plan, if that is okay with you?"

"Sure. Will that help with the pain in my chest?"

"It might, but in the meantime, I would like you to take more hydromorphone for the pain," he explained.

"I don't like taking that stuff," Jim confessed.

"Why not?"

"Well, I don't want to get addicted. I've heard all these stories."

"Mr. Schreuders, you will not get addicted. It will help with your pain. It's okay for you to take it. We will also get you in for a CT scan if that is okay with you?"

"Yes, that's good, thank you. Can I go home now?" Jim asked again.

"You don't live in London, do you?" he asked while looking back at his paperwork. "The CT scan will be done in a day or two. I thought you could just stay here till then."

"I want to go home. Can I just go and come back tomorrow for the CT?"

"Sure, if you are comfortable doing that, then it's fine with me," he agreed. Both looked my way, the doctor questioningly while Jim pleaded with his eyes.

"He wants to go home, so I can do that if you are okay with it," I shrugged. It was agreed that I would take Jim home, and we would return whenever the CT was scheduled.

After the doctor took his leave, Nathan stayed for a few minutes to talk to us about the meeting.

"What do you think? You didn't ask any questions," Jim asked him.

"It is what it is. I was just there to listen," he softly said.

Once Nathan left, I helped Jim dress and pack his belongings to come home with me. Having mismatched his shirt buttons, I came in front of him to do them for him. While concentrating on tying one of the buttons, he took my hands and looked down into my eyes.

"I'm sorry for making you drive back again with me tomorrow. I just can't stay here. I had horrible nightmares last night. This room is so small, and I feel stuffed back here. It is so out of the way. It's lonely and depressing. I just want to be in bed beside you. I just need to get out of here," he said sadly.

"I get it. I have no problem bringing you back. I love you," I said, and kissed him. "Sleeping is better with you in my bed, too," I smiled up at him before grabbing the rest of his bags and leaving the hospital hand in hand.

A few days later, and nineteen months after his first diagnosis with Dr. Ferguson, they called us to come for a CT scan in London. While we were there, they were making time to do more tattoos if Jim needed them for the upcoming radiation Jim had agreed to do. He encouraged me to come with him to see how far they would let me go. To our surprise, I was able to go right into the room where they were going to do the CT scan and check his breathing. After discussing when to start radiation and the best timeframe, he mentioned he would still like to work in the mornings if possible. They would let us know, promising to do their best to get the time Jim wanted. A nurse led me to a small consultation room with three comfy chairs. I took the chair closest to the door and read my book while I waited. I only read a few pages before I heard Jim and a nurse joking in the hallway.

"Jim, you can wait here with your wife. The doctor will be here shortly to talk with you both," she smiled.

"Thank you," we said in unison.

After taking the seat to my left, I turned to him, "That was quick."

"They can use the tattoos I had last time, so I didn't need to get more," he smiled. A few minutes later, Dr. Palmer walked in and introduced himself. Seeing the Dutch sweatshirt Jim wore, he commented on it, telling us he did some of his studies in the Netherlands.

"We doctors have a saying," he smiled. "If a Dutch farmer comes in with pain, he is having a heart attack because that is the only thing that will bring a stubborn Dutch farmer in to see a doctor." We laughed together, knowing that this is so true for those we know. He then moved the conversation to Jim. "I have talked with Dr. Fortin, Dr. Lang, Dr. Logan, and two other doctors about your care, Jim. We think radiation is the best course of action for your cancer at this time. We would like to start you out with fifteen sessions. It should stop the tumours from bleeding and maybe even shrink them a little. But we want you to understand that it will not stop it completely. This is just to buy you some more time. How much? We do not know." He then went through some more information, and we were given more papers to read about the radiation, which looked much like the previous paperwork. Dr. Palmer's upbeat, friendly manner set us at ease to the point where we, too, could joke around amid the seriousness of it all. He finished by telling us he wanted to start soon. Were we okay with starting on Monday? He was sure they could figure it all out by then, even if they had to work double time on it.

Decisions

THE NEXT DAY we made our way to Stratford to pick out our new bed. Unlike Goldilocks, the first bed was just right but sadly delivery would take six months due to COVID. We couldn't wait that long. The second bed was the Cadillac version of beds. It had two remotes for the two separate mattresses, under glow to see where you were walking in the night, and vibrators for your head and for your feet. I must admit that brought a round of giggles out of us which abruptly stopped when the salesman gave us the Cadillac price. Off we went to see the last bed. It didn't take us long to see that this last bed was not good quality. We decided to go home and think about it.

The next morning, we made our way back to London to meet with Dr. Fortin to see if surgery was still an option on the table. Even though we talked to Dr. Palma, who had already told us it wasn't, Jim needed to hear it from Dr. Fortin herself.

As we waited for her in the large room again, we listened to other patients' conversations and surfed the web with the hospital's free Wi-Fi, trying to pass the time. When our number was called, we followed a nice gentleman who brought us to Dr. Fortin's tiny consultation room. When she finally arrived, she turned to the young man working with her.

"You see this gentleman. Do you know what he was doing after two weeks of surgery?"

"I have no idea," said the student.

"Mr. Schreuders here was out driving his motorcycle and had a little accident," she said, shaking her head. Jim beamed with pleasure as she remembered him. She then asked him how he was otherwise. She was very patient with us as we asked many questions during our long meeting. Jim finally came right out and asked her if she could do surgery to get the mets out.

Point blank she said, "No." Then she continued. "Jim, I could go in and take stuff out. I would be up for the challenge, and I could get lots out. But it would be major surgery, and your quality of life wouldn't be good after that." She explained that surgery would have them taking a big chunk of his lung and some other organ parts to get the required margin. After that, he would have to have a major recovery time.

"You will not be comfortable and most likely spend most of it in the hospital, which you have already said you don't want to do. I don't think that is the answer here. We have done surgeries like that in the past but have learned from them. We now know our patients will have a better life without it." Jim and I could see her point and agreed with her.

"I think it is time for you to talk to Dr. Logan. I think they were booking an appointment for you," she said while leafing through her papers.

"Yes, we have an appointment," I said.

"I want you to understand that drug therapy does not stop this type of cancer, but it has the possibility of slowing it down. But I will leave that to Dr. Logan. She can better explain that all to you as it is her expertise, not mine," she advised.

We then discussed Jim's pain. He was taking 2 mg of hydromorphone for the pain whenever he felt it coming on. This pain came regularly. She gave him another prescription for a longer lasting 3 mg pill that he could take. If he still had pain, he was to take the 2 mg one as well.

As we came to the end of our appointment, Jim calmly told her about being frustrated when no one was willing to give him answers about the blood in his lungs. She apologized for that, thinking they figured we would be seeing her today, and she would explain it to us. But she was not sure, and she understood Jim's frustration and apologized once again. She pulled out a business card from her pocket. She put her personal number on it, telling us to call her if there was any confusion about the plan or anxiety related to the uncertainty. She was very willing to try to help us, and we confirmed I would call her office Monday morning and let her know how the new longer-lasting meds were working.

"Oh, before we go, can I get a note for work?" Jim asked.

Looking at him for the count of ten before saying, "Okay, I will be the one to put it out there. Someone has to. If you have six to twelve months left to live, do you want to be spending that at work or with your family?" she boldly stated.

"I enjoy my work."

"He really does. It's like his other family," I added, trying to help her understand. But deep down, wanting to argue her point more.

"Well, you have to figure out what is most important to you and what you want to be doing with the time you have left," she kindly said, turning back to the computer. She typed up a note that indicated he would be off work indefinitely. Leaving to get the letter off the printer, I started collecting our coats, water bottles and my purse. When she returned, handing Jim the letter, we said our goodbyes and sincerely thanked her for all of her help. As we slowly headed down the hall, Jim reached out for my hand; I smiled up at him as we headed out of the hospital.

On the way home we discussed the appointment. The conversation was interspersed with periods of silence, each of us in our own thoughts. I couldn't hold it in anymore. I told Jim I was a little frustrated about the thought of possibly having to share him with those at his work.

"We always talked about spending time with grandkids and going for motorcycle rides in our retirement years. Can we not take this time off work and think that way? Can we enjoy the time we have left as our retirement years, instead of pushing to return to work?" I pleaded.

"I'll think about it," he thoughtfully said, as I prayed for the time we had left together.

At one point on our way home, my phone rang, and it was the gentleman who offered to buy us a bed. After a discussion on our findings the day before, he arranged to buy the Cadillac bed.

We didn't know what to think or how to feel. This was a *huge* gift. Not only in monetary value, but as a gift of time—we could still be together through the nights. We could lie next to each other, hear each other breathing—or snoring—and hold tight for just a little bit longer. We were each other's best friend. To us, our relationship was worth far more than any "thing."

Christmas Gifts

WITH OUR FAMILY Christmas just two days later, Jim and I decided we would stay home to watch the service online, allowing Jim to nap before the festivities. It was agreed that Joshua would stay with us while the rest of the kids went to church in person. Since Jim's health was unpredictable, our oldest, Derek, and his wife, Danielle, offered to host Christmas at their house. This seemed like a good solution, as they live down the street from us. Jim could slip out for a nap in his chair if he needed rest, and return to enjoy the festivities later. After the service, Jim pushed his chair back into the reclining position and soon fell asleep. I went upstairs to finish wrapping my special gift for Jim. I would give it to him later when we were with all the grandkids. After only a few minutes I thought I heard Joshua talking to someone downstairs. Waiting for him to call me, I hurriedly finished wrapping. When I came down the stairs, no one was at the door; but there were two huge boxes of food on the bench beside the door. Hunting for Joshua, and finding him sprawled out on the couch across from Jim's recliner, I asked who was at the door.

"There you are! I didn't know where you went," he whispered, trying not to wake Dad. "I do not know them, but they said they were part of the homeschool group and went to the church where Victoria's office is in. They said the food is from their church." He got up and went with me to the boxes. There was a Christmas dinner for our *whole* family in those boxes! Right down to the cranberry sauce, gravy and pumpkin pie. Along with some grocery cards. Tears flowed down my cheeks as I had him help me put the meat in the freezer and the fresh veggies in the fridge. Jim stirred from the commotion coming from the kitchen. Stretching, he asked what was going on. Shock registered on his face when I told him what happened, while the kids came in from church, getting what they needed before heading to Derek's.

Jim's phone dinged with a message. It was my pen pal, Wilma, and her husband Jan, from Holland. Wilma and I started writing when we were ten years old. I went to

Holland to meet her in person for the first time when I was eighteen. The next year she and her now husband came for our wedding, as Wilma would be one of my bridesmaids. Jim and I were finally able to visit them in 2018 after having stayed in touch for twenty-nine years. All four of us had an unbelievable ten-day visit. It was not uncommon to have a video call as they were requesting now. So once the kids all left, with the message that we would be right over when we finished the call, we set up the laptop and got comfy on the couch with Jim's arm protectively around me.

"Hey! How are you guys?" Jan asked.

"Ja, ik ben good," Jim said in his sparse Dutch with a huge smile.

Laughing, Jan asked if Jim had received his email.

"No. You sent me an email?" Jim said, leaning ahead to pick up his phone from the coffee table beside the laptop.

"Yes, you look at it later. We talk now," Jan said as he started talking about the weather both here and there and Jan's business that he runs over there. Then they inquired about Jim's health.

"We want to come to visit you, Jim and Joanne," he said, shocking us.

"We would love to have you, but I don't know what to say. If I end up in the hospital, I want Joanne with me, and you wouldn't be able to visit us. That seems like a waste of money on a plane ticket." Jim sadly explained.

"Well, we will leave it up to you. We really want to come to visit you. You just say when and we will come, next week, next month, three months from now. You just tell us what is good for you. You think about it," he encouraged. We could tell this was important to them too.

"We will talk about it and see what we can do," Jim said thoughtfully. I was excited but also frustrated because, as Jim said, our lives were in the air. From one day to the next, we didn't know what God had in store for us. Saying our farewells with the promise to keep them informed, we checked Jim's email from Jan. As we read, we could see that they were serious about coming, even if it meant on short notice. Tucking that information in the back of our minds, we grabbed what we needed and headed out the door to Derek's house.

Once there, we headed to the living room to spend time with the youngest grandkids while the older ones helped Aunt Melissa build their annual gingerbread contest entry. The other couples were already spreading out their candy and tracing out the gingerbread patterns they had made on the sheets of gingerbread Desiree had made beforehand for me. Jim got himself down on the floor with some of the grandsons, watching the train go round and round under the Christmas tree.

After a while, Jim lay on the couch to rest. I asked him if he needed me to bring him home. He assured me the couch would be fine for now. Again, I was amazed at how he has always been able to sleep with people around, remembering our own kids climbing on him while he slept.

As the gingerbread houses came together, I started taking photos of the finished products to put on Facebook for the annual judging. I smiled as I watched the two newest additions, the young men who were dating our daughters, get right into the gingerbread contest.

As the gingerbread remains were being cleaned up, I asked the grandkids to come into the living room with me to give Papa his present. Jim looked at me quizzically as I handed him a flat, wrapped gift with a smaller box wrapped separately on top. Inside the small box, he found a small camera for him to hang up in his chicken house that he could connect to his phone with an app. This way, he could watch his precious chickens no matter where he was. Laughing, he turned to the flat gift while the grandkids stood close, some trying to help him open it. Inside, he found a child's book I had made with Shutterfly. Laughing, he read the title aloud, "Papa's Chickens by Joanne Schreuders." Opening it up, he started to read silently. I told him it was a book he had to read to the grandkids. So, starting over, with the grandkids surrounding him, he read aloud. "Once upon a time, there was a Papa." As he turned the pages, we heard Parker's little excited voice, "Hey, that's me! Chloe, that's you!" Then, as the other kids started pointing out who was who, Papa had to stop and settle everyone for a minute. As he continued, he laughed as the book began with the photos of Crispy and continued with the chickens he has now. Melissa and I had even gone out one night when Jim was at his men's bible study and taken pictures with sparklers and a strobe light. "Party in the house!" Everyone laughed as we enjoyed the book together.

After a delicious meal together, we sat and visited while the grandkids ran off the sugar-high from the gingerbread candy. As they started to crash, the families started to head for home, each trying to leave their edible structures behind. Yes, behind. Who wants the temptation of all that candy looking at you each and every day?

The following day, before Jim started his next radiation session, he emailed payroll with the letter from the lung surgeon, to say he would be off work indefinitely. He also let them know that his last *full* day of work was eleven days earlier, but a few days before that he was in the hospital. Not knowing what they wanted him to do, he offered to sit down and figure out which days he had worked and which he hadn't worked. He received a reply that they would figure it out, and he was not to worry about it. They also told him about the long-term disability available through work and emailed that information to him. With that dealt with, he prepared for his next radiation session later that day.

Our friend Ed picked up Jim and took him for the radiation while I stayed behind to prepare our room for our new beds. The young delivery men set them up, making sure they hooked everything up correctly. They tried the vibrator button, and the bed loudly moved across the wood floor.

"It shouldn't be so bad with the mattress on it," he said to me with a chuckle. Shortly after they left, I wondered why I made the beds as I watched everyone take turns climbing into them and trying out the new remotes.

"You better not mix up the remotes in the middle of the night and move my bed," Jim declared. We laughed at all the possibilities of comical errors these beds could cause. (Just for the record, I didn't mean to push the foot vibrator button on the remote in the middle of the night, startling Jim into an upright position.)

"Who gave you the beds?" the kids asked.

"We were asked not to say," we answered, taking this as a teaching moment.

"Why?"

"They did it to help us out. Not to say, 'Look what I did.' They wanted to be Jesus's hands and feet. Helping others is what God wants us to do without looking for praise from the people around us."

"Don't they want to be thanked?"

"God knows what they have done, and that's the most important thing. Not what others around us think." They went off pondering this.

Think about it

Have you ever helped someone or given someone a gift without them knowing who it was from? Others do not need to see what you have done. What really matters is that God knows. He sees all things. *"But when you give to the needy, do not let your left hand know what your right hand is doing, so that your giving may be in secret. Then your Father, who sees what is done in secret will reward you"* (Matthew 6:3–4).

In the meantime, we received an email from the lady at Jim's work with the information for long-term disability. She also told us that they would be paying Jim right up until his last day of work, December 9, and not to worry about the previous days he missed. Shocked and slightly taken aback, Jim sent a grateful reply.

The fifteen aggressive radiation treatments started on December 20 and would continue on the 21st, 22nd, and 23rd. At the second session, they told Jim the radiologist wanted him not to skip so many days during Christmas. They would be coming in to give him his treatment on the 24th and the 27th. Coming in a bit early, as was his rule, they still had to start up the machines.

"Do you have other patients today?" he asked the technologist.

"Nope, you are the only one. As soon as we are done, I shut it all down and go back home again." Well, that made us feel important.

On the morning of the 26th, Jim came in from the chicken coop after feeding the chickens and showed off his very first egg! After debating with himself, he decided to fry it up for breakfast before preparing to watch church online. Again, he said his head was cloudy and that he felt a little confused. Tucking that information in the back of my mind, we went on with our day.

Following church, we had Christmas with our kids who still lived at home. We laughed at the gifts the girls bought for us. "The University of Guelph Dad (and Mom)" t-shirts from Melissa and "Brock University Dad (and Mom)" sweatshirts from Elly. Jim gave me two gifts; one was a beautiful necklace, and the second was a charm for my charm bracelet. I looked down at the dime-sized charm with a single letter "J" on it.

Swallowing hard, he said, "It's a J for Joanne." Tears glistened in our eyes as we quickly looked away from each other.

Looking at the charm again, I said quietly for only him to hear, "It's a J for Jim," and I shyly peeked up at him. He gave a weak smile, not disagreeing.

As Jim continued radiation treatment, we received the news that we had a new granddaughter, Sophia Marie, daughter to Christina and Cody. This kept Jim in good spirits as the radiation was becoming more difficult to deal with. By the eighth treatment, on Thursday, Jim's pain started to be more localized on the radiation sight. He didn't think he could make it into the vehicle for the one-hour drive to London, but he did. All the while, I tried to avoid all the manholes and went slowly over five railroad tracks while we both gritted our teeth. These roads were desperately in need of construction! Once at the hospital, we were able to talk to a doctor who informed us that the pain was from the radiation swelling. We doubled all his pain meds and gave him a five-day steroid for swelling. Now that he had a hard time going to the radiation appointments by himself, we got permission for me to go in with him as his caregiver. He now needed me to help him get his jacket, sweatshirt, and boots off and on.

The weekend was good. He seemed to be improving. He even stayed up to celebrate the New Year on Friday with some friends and family here at home. We prayed for a miracle and for Jim to have a chance to hold his new granddaughter.

During the holiday break, Nathan came over and helped hook up Jim's Christmas gift, the "chicken" monitor, in his chicken condo. Finding a good spot on the ceiling of the condo, he mounted the camera. With the camera connected to an app on his phone, Jim could now see his "girls" any time of day as they went in and out of the small chicken door. Not only could he see them, but he could hear them and talk to them too. A man and his gadgets, what can I say? He was happy, and that's all that mattered to me.

Palliative Care Talk

SUNDAY MORNING, AFTER a good sleep, Jim got up and made a bacon and egg breakfast for himself and me. As I did every morning, I asked him how he was feeling. He said he had a little pain. Thinking he would feel a bit better if he stood in the hot shower, he took his towel and headed in that direction. After he came out, as I was helping put his socks on for him, I could see that he was still uncomfortable. Informing me that he was going to check on his chickens, he slowly made his way through the living room, slipped his boots and coat on in the mudroom, and headed outside. I watched through the kitchen window and saw him slowly trudge by in the snow as he walked a little more than the length of the house to get to the "Chicken Condo." By the time he made it back, after stopping to put the handful of eggs in the fridge, I could see he had pain etched on his face. He sat in his comfy chair, ready to watch the church service with us. The recliner just was not comfy enough this morning. He got up in tears as the pain just got worse.

The kids and I were watching Dad, feeling helpless. Our church family began singing about God's breath being in our lungs—the song "Great Are You Lord" by David Leonard, Jason Ingram, and Leslie Jordon.[6] But we were all having a hard time concentrating on the online service.

I followed Jim and made a phone call to the emergency department at St. Marys, then to the radiology hotline in London. Jim climbed back into bed, hoping to relieve some pain. I finally messaged our doctor, and we decided that I should call for an ambulance to take him to St. Marys hospital. Jim's pain was now excruciating.

The ambulance arrived, backing into the snowy driveway. I directed them in through the living room patio door. I led them through the house to where Jim lay moaning in bed, with the church service still playing on the other side of the wall. The

---

[6] David Leonard, Jason Ingram, Leslie Jordan, "Great Are You Lord," Integrity's Alleluia Music, 2012. .

kids were sitting there watching but not listening to the sermon. After a quick assessment, Jim said he could sit on the chair they had, and they transported him out to the living room where the stretcher waited. I texted Victoria asking her to come to sit with the kids. Then I told them I would be back as soon as possible. Victoria messaged to say she was on her way. I knew they were old enough to be left alone, but they would need more family to surround them.

When I returned to the living room, Derek stood in the mudroom doorway.

"Danielle was driving past and saw the ambulance. She turned right around and came back to tell me. I came right over," he explained.

"Do you have a ride to the hospital?" The paramedic asked me.

"I'll drive behind you with my car," I said, looking down at my shaking hands.

"I'll drive her," Derek told the paramedic, and relief washed over me. I felt the tension release just a little.

"I think that would be for the best," he said, while they finished strapping Jim in and taking him through the snow to the ambulance.

Climbing into the truck beside Derek, a few tears ran down my cheeks; I swiped them away. I felt so small and helpless sitting next to my oldest son. We talked about what had transpired in the past few days as we started down the road. Less than fifteen minutes later we arrived at the hospital. Derek pulled up to the door and let me out while promising to check on his siblings.

Once the paramedics got Jim situated in a room, I was allowed to join him. A smiling lady came to take his blood after the nurse gave him some more "happy juice." This is what we called his liquid morphine. God had encouraged me to message Karen, a friend who had been in the hospital many times throughout her life. She would give me her "Cole's notes" summary of various medications, and help me ask the doctor and nurses the right questions about possible medications. After another X-ray, they decided to book him in for an emergency CT scan at Stratford hospital. Pumped with morphine, he said he would be fine to go with me in the truck to the hospital. We called home and asked the girls to bring the truck for us. As we were ready to leave, we realized we needed to swing by the house to pick up Jim's coat and boots. In the meantime, the nurse gave Jim an extra pair of hospital socks which I helped him put on before pulling the truck around to the emergency door, out of the snow. After the CT scan at the Stratford hospital, we went back to St. Marys, and I tucked Jim back in the bed he was in before. At this time, there was a shift change for the doctor, and we were pleased to see our own family doctor, Dr. Thornton, on the floor. She called London for their opinion about the scans and bloodwork. They reported back that it was just the radiation doing its job.

Dr. Thornton came in to have a good discussion with us. She told us that the emergency department was empty, and we ended up talking for nearly an hour, uninterrupted, about Jim's condition and care.

"Jim, most people think palliative care is the end of life. In reality, palliative care is keeping the patient comfortable while following their wishes. I have had patients in palliative care who get well and don't need it anymore. It is a way to get things in place in your home, so that you don't have to make trips to the hospital amid pain like you did today. An example would be setting you up for in-home care, where a doctor and nurses would visit your home to see you. Also, we would get a Symptom Response Kit in your home for medications and things for the nurses to use to administer any medications you might need. Would you agree to this?"

"If I don't have to go through that pain again, and then travel by ambulance, that would be nice," he said.

At this time she asked if we would allow her to be on Jim's palliative care team. She wanted to be his palliative care doctor. To which we both answered with a resounding, "Yes, please!"

"Jim, I think the other doctors talked to you already about the Province of Ontario "Do Not Resuscitate" form? I want to take a minute to tell you my story. My Dad had lung cancer, and he didn't sign the paper. Like you, he wanted to stay alive. When the time came, he was resuscitated and later regretted it. His quality of life was not good, and there were all kinds of other problems. He had wished he had signed the paper. I need to tell you that if you are resuscitated, then you will need to have an intubating tube. Due to the nature of your disease, this tube will not be removed," she quietly said to Jim with regret in her eyes.

"I'm just not ready yet," he said sadly.

"I understand, Jim. When you are ready, you need to tell your home care nurse and me, as well as your family. You also have to remember that this is hard on your family. When you decide, they don't have to. You have to keep them informed of your wishes. You will also want to look into the disability tax credit and critical illness insurance."

Like every visit, COVID came into the conversation, "Have you had all your shots yet, Jim?" Jim explained his heart issues after the last two COVID shots. She promised to look into it.

"Should I be having my booster shot?" I asked, "Will it affect whether or not I can go to the hospital or doctor appointments with Jim?"

"She has to come with me. I need her help," Jim urged.

"Yes, it would probably be for the best if she did. I am working at the COVID clinic, so I can set something up. I'll have my receptionist book something for you,

Joanne. Do any of the kids need their shots too?" She told us that we needed to stay away from people at this stage in the game. At least for a month, to see where the numbers go with COVID cases. She told us the kids needed to stay home from school and do it online. The schools were a petri dish full of germs Jim didn't need. We were sad as that meant we couldn't see our older kids or grandkids as they all had someone either in school or daycare. We reassured ourselves that we could do this for a month. One month was doable, right?

After going through everything she would do for us—registering him for Stratford's palliative care team, looking into his COVID shots, getting him stronger pain meds, making sure I would keep track of when and how much medication to give him and recording his pain level on a scale of 0–10—she left to write out the prescription. We left a bit later with the prescription in hand and felt reassured that we were in good hands. We both sighed in relief. We knew God had a plan. He had been walking with us and was already ahead of us. We prayed for complete healing, and for peace if complete healing was not in his plan. Our God is a Great God, the Great Physician and a miracle worker, whom we love with all our heart, soul, mind, and strength.

That night I found a little brown notebook that I could use to start recording Jim's daily vitals and meds. There was so much to remember and I needed one place to keep all the information. This book would be handy and would go wherever Jim went.

Monday was filled with mixed emotions. Christina came to visit with our newest granddaughter Sophia. We had wanted to travel to Mount Forest to meet her earlier, but it would have been too much for Jim.

"Meet your new grandbaby, Papa," Christina said, handing her to Jim as he sat in his recliner. Jim, all smiles, gently took her in his arms, cradling her as tears sprang from his eyes and his lip quivered.

"Hi, little Sophia. I'm your Papa," he said, looking down at her sweet five-day-old face. The rest of us looked on in silence. A small sob escaped his lips as he cradled her tightly, nervously rearranging the pink blanket around her. Tears escaped the eyes of everyone in the room as we wondered if this would be the last time he would hold her. Christina stepped closer to her dad, squeezing his arm.

"We love you, Papa," she whispered shakily, going down to give him an awkward hug. He smiled up at her through glistening eyes, unable to speak. We left Papa to sit quietly with sleeping Sophia, whispering to her and praying over her.

Pain

THE NEXT DAY, Tuesday, we received a phone call from Community Care Services. They had received the referral from Dr. Thornton and were wondering if Jim could come into the office or if they needed to make a house call. Jim felt he could drive there, so we didn't have to put anyone out. I, on the other hand, thought he would be more comfortable at home. But Jim arranged for us to go to Stratford on Saturday to meet with Jessica to discuss his care.

Jim, having dragged himself out of bed on both Tuesday and now Wednesday, he tried yet again to make the painstakingly brutal trip to the hospital for radiation treatment. When we got to the hospital, Jim was asking for the plastic baggie with his "just in case" meds—Long-lasting hydromorphone, breakthrough hydromorphone, Tylenol extra strength, and Tums. I was starting to feel like a drug dealer, hoping I could keep them all straight. He could barely walk on these two days because of the pain. He would make it to the double doors of the clinic entrance and then willingly sit in a wheelchair. I knew it was bad because he didn't fight me or say, "I can do it!" which he had in the past.

On Wednesday afternoon, as I sat in waiting room three, reading the book I kept in my purse for such occasions, I was surprised to see Jim come around the corner in his wheelchair, pushed by his nurse

"That was quick today," I said.

"I don't feel good," he quietly told me after the nurse left him in my care. "I feel like they just cranked it way up and gave me all they had." He looked awful. Slowly we worked at getting his sweatshirt and jacket on. I tried to pull up his slip-on work boots, but he hardly had the energy to push his foot down. He sat slumped in the wheelchair as I slowly and quietly pushed him down the halls, back to the main waiting room, and up to registration to get his next day appointment, all the while wondering if he would make it. When we reached the door, he ripped off his mask; he just

103

needed air. I offered to bring the truck around, but he thought he could make it, as we had parked close to the door. Partway to the truck we stopped at the park bench so he could rest. Again I offered to bring the truck closer.

"Just give me a minute. I need to keep moving," he tried to reassure me. Finally, making it to the truck, I helped him in and buckled his seatbelt. Going around the truck, I climbed behind the wheel and we headed for home. I wanted to stop at the grocery store on the way home, but I could see he was grimacing with each bump in the road. I decided stopping would be a bad idea. Getting home was the goal. Once there, he went straight to his chair and slept.

A few weeks before, I had talked to a lady at the bank about remortgaging the house. After some delay due to vacations on her end, we had an appointment booked for this afternoon. Knowing Jim wouldn't make it, I called the bank and explained our situation. I then asked if I could pick up the paperwork, get Jim to sign it, and bring it back. They agreed to this and we were able to renew our mortgage for another five years at the same low weekly payment, which made paying our bills more doable.

Later that night, Dr. Thornton called about Jim's COVID shots. Jim didn't think it was worth it at this point due to his declining health.

On Thursday we woke up and I was going to start getting ready to take him to his next appointment.

"I can't go. I don't feel good. I feel like they gave it all they had yesterday. I can't do this anymore. Can you call and tell them I'm done?" he said, letting out a little moan from where he lay in the bed. I sat beside him, combing his hair back with my fingers. Quietly sitting there, I didn't know what to do. What was the right answer? I knew this was too much for him. I could see the pain he was in.

"You are sure?" I double-checked.

"Yes, I can't do this anymore," he mumbled, trying to relax. I reached for my cell phone and called the clinic, telling them he wouldn't be in today for his treatment. They asked about his symptoms and tried to make sure he was okay. I was surprised at how easy it was to cancel, as I had prepared myself for pushback. Before hanging up, they gave me the time for his appointment the next day, and I dutifully wrote it down on my calendar. All the while I was praying that God would take away his pain. Again, he spent the day in his chair, and I did his chicken chores.

Friday was a repeat of the day before. I knew then that we were done. Being bolder this day, I told them we wouldn't be coming back. While he lay in bed, I formulated an email for the kids to let them know what was going on. Shortly after sending it, Derek called to talk to Jim while he lay in bed, unable to get to his chair.

"Come on, Dad, you are almost done. You can finish this."

"Derek, I'm done. I just can't," he said, sadly.

"But you only have three more to do, Dad," he urged.

"Derek, I'm sorry. I'm not giving up. I just can't do any more of this radiation. I just can't." Jim felt that his children didn't understand, thinking he was giving up, but he knew he just couldn't do it anymore.

"Okay, Dad. I just thought if you needed a push, I would do that for you," he said, backing down. "As long as you are sure?"

"Yes, I'm sure," he said through his weakness. We had to accept the reality; any further radiation was too painful. The kids who were isolated at home with us could see this, unlike our married kids who couldn't see him. The doctors were still trying to work Jim's pain meds to the point of comfort but hadn't succeeded yet.

Later that morning, after helping him get up for the day, I noticed Jim's colour was not good. It seemed he was turning more grey in colour each day and getting more confused. This morning, he was going to take a shower but didn't know which way the bathroom was. You could see this bothered him. Something was not right. While I waited for him to finish showering—I now needed to help him dress—I messaged our family doctor, now our palliative care doctor. I let her know that he looked grey and that he was confused. His pain was seven out of ten for most of the day. He also seemed close to losing his voice over the past week. He couldn't talk loudly, which the kids joked about. She messaged back and said I should take him to the hospital to get looked at. When he was dressed, he was exhausted and still in pain. I told him that the doctor wanted him to go to the hospital. She even said I was to call the ambulance if he couldn't go in our vehicle. Back in bed again, he chose the ambulance.

I went to the kids in the next room to explain that the doctor wanted Dad to go to the hospital and that I was going to call the ambulance. Trying to put their minds at ease, I explained that it was not an emergency; it was just the most comfortable way for Dad to get there. I made sure they knew what was for dinner and gave instructions for cooking it. When they finished asking their questions, which I sometimes didn't feel capable of answering, I called the ambulance. While waiting, I grabbed a few snacks for my purse and photocopied the page in my notebook where I had written the meds he had already taken today and at what times. When the new ambulance drivers arrived, I showed them in and reviewed the information they needed. I drove myself behind the ambulance, as this time I was more calm than the last time.

Dr. Thornton had called ahead, informing the doctor on-call about Jim's case. When Jim arrived at the hospital, he was immediately put in his own room because he had a cough, a symptom of COVID. They did a COVID test and sent it off for results, which would take at least three days. The doctor did the routine check-up, listening to his lungs and asking a million and one questions that had become routine for us.

It almost made us want to roll our eyes but we knew they were just doing their job. In the end, we learned that Jim was toxic. His body was not processing the hydromorphone as it should. They would flush out his system and change his medication to actual morphine.

"What's the difference between hydromorphone and morphine? Why didn't they start him on morphine?" I asked the doctor.

"Hydromorphone is synthetic and is more condensed than morphine. It's usually what we start with," he explained, turning to Jim. "So, we will start you on an IV and get you to a room. You will have to stay here for a few days until we can get you on the right track." Jim, still a little confused, agreed. I followed a bit later as they wheeled him to his new room. As the porter pushed him through the door, she turned to me and said I was not allowed in because he was in quarantine. I stepped in anyway, kissing him and telling him I would be back in the morning. Turning, I left Jim behind yet again.

"Good morning, lover! Is your mind clearer?" I texted the following morning at 8:00 am.

"Yes, a little," he answered. I could tell he was not in the mood for conversation, so I kept it short, telling him I would be there around lunchtime. Nathan came over with his young son Darius, who was bundled up in his snowsuit. They came to help bring wood to the house from the pile in the yard so we could stay warm. Calvin and Joshua pulled it in from outside as he brought it to the door. I stuck my head out and waved to Darius, talking to him for a few minutes while he sat in the snow a good distance away. I hated these COVID rules. Would our grandkids grow up knowing how much we loved them?

At 11:20 am, I received a text from Jim: "The kids are texting me to see how I am. I just don't know what to say anymore." Followed by another, "Are you coming?" I could hear the sadness in his words. I finished what I was doing and went to him.

I walked into the room and saw his face light up. His colour was improving, and he was more alert than yesterday. He was so glad to see me. He was frustrated that they were keeping him in isolation due to his cough, knowing it was from the tumours in his lungs, not from COVID. I sat with him for a few minutes before a nurse came by and got mad at me because I was not suited up. Apologizing, I asked her to show me what I needed to do. Well, they had a cart outside his bedroom door. I needed a yellow disposable gown and a blue mask for my mouth and nose. Then I needed to put on a face shield, which caused my glasses to fog up. Then, and only then, was I allowed to enter Jim's room. I entered cautiously as my glasses wouldn't allow me to go faster. While I attempted to find the chair, Jim's snicker turned to laughter.

"Will you take that silly thing off your face? You can't even see where you are going." I did, but I kept it close. We discussed how ridiculous it was since I was with him the whole time at home. If he had COVID, then I should have it too. But we were not going to make a fuss, or they might not let me in at all.

I could tell he was still sad. We talked about a variety of things that afternoon, but mostly how he wanted to do this well. He wanted to tie up anything that was left loose. He wanted to make things right if they were not. In particular, he had been bothered lately by some past things with his parents. He felt he hadn't been the best son he could have been. I could see it bothered him, as he, in his mind, wanted to make it right. He felt like he needed to ask for forgiveness, but he didn't know how much time he had and if he would see them again. I encouraged him to call them and get it off his chest; I could see the weight of it hanging on him. He did just that. He called his mom, who put him on speakerphone for Dad to listen in. He asked for forgiveness, which was given amid tears and affirmation of their love. It was a beautiful thing to witness.

The next morning, after Jim texted to remind me to do chicken chores, I replied and said I hadn't forgotten and would do it in a minute. He assured me he was not rushing me; he just wanted to make sure they were not forgotten. I bundled up and made my way out there. It was so nice to be out in the fresh January air, not in the house or a hospital. I lingered a little before entering the chicken condo.

I fed and watered the chickens and was about to put my hand in the nesting box when I heard, "Bok! Bok! Don't steal my eggs Mrs. Schreuders," scaring me half to death.

"Jim!" I reprimanded as I heard a chuckle over the monitor speaker. We had a little chat out there among the hungry chickens before I headed back into the house with a smile on my face. I thanked the Lord that Jim's sense of humour was returning.

Later that morning I brought the laptop to the hospital so we could watch church online together. I had also brought some mail and cards for him to look at. A young man, Daniel, one of Jim's cadets, along with his family, had made a DVD for Jim to watch. We popped the DVD into the laptop and watched. They wished him well, each one using one of their talents in music or reading a story for Jim. Jim just loved the farming stop-action Lego movie Daniel had made for him.

A while later, the doctor came in to talk to us about Jim's new medication. Apparently, when they started him on the 10 mg of morphine Jim's heart started to race.

"I felt like I had to hold my heart in my chest, or it would have come right out," he explained to the doctor.

"Yeah, so you most likely had too much morphine," he apologized. "We will start you on 5 mg and see how you do with that."

"Can I go home now?" he asked.

"Well, I think maybe you should stay here till we get your meds figured out," he suggested.

"I think I need to go home. I can't walk the halls or go anywhere because they think I might have COVID because of this cough I came in with. I walk to this chair two steps from the bed, then take three steps to the bathroom, and back to the bed. My bum is sore. At least if I go home, I can walk around more. As for the meds, just don't give me 10 mg, and I will be fine," he reasoned.

The doctor was thinking. He turned to me, "Are you okay with him coming home without trying the new dose of meds?"

"Yes, she is," Jim said, seeing an opening and eager to go home.

"I guess. If he feels it will be okay," I shrugged to the doctor, feeling just a little stuck between a rock and a hard place.

"Okay then, but let us know if there are any problems. Or let your palliative care nurses know," he sternly said to Jim.

Meanwhile, I got a call from Nathan. Darius was beside himself because he didn't get to see Papa yesterday. He wondered where we were in the little St. Marys hospital just down the road from his house. After confirming that he was not allowed in, I told him what window we were at but explained that we were leaving soon. So, they made their way over. The windows on this side of the hospital were high, so Nathan grabbed Darius's snowsuit and heaved him up above his head. Darius waved and talked to Papa through the hospital window while perched on his Dad's palm, brightening each other's day.

By late afternoon Jim was back at home. Tucked in his reclining chair beside the wood stove, he was complaining about his bum still being so sore. Before bed that night we discovered he had bedsores. This made sense to us, considering the time he spent this past week sitting in his chair and bed at home and then in the hospital. It slowly healed over the coming days while we treated it with polysporin; the nurses warned us he would now be more susceptible to these sores.

I now had the trusty brown notebook that stayed with him wherever he went. The date was on the top of each page, with the time he took his required meds listed underneath. I also listed his pain level at the time of each med. On the side of the page, in a box, we wrote his vitals in the morning and again in the evening. I had to take his temperature, heart rate, oxygen levels and blood pressure morning and night. On the bottom of the page, I would note any appointments we were to have that day and any questions we needed to ask a doctor or the home nurse. Once I asked the question, I could even write the answers down—it was getting too hard to remember everything. I thought I had a lot of meds to remember before, but now…

- Ibuprofen 400 mg 3x/day for seven days (for pain)
- Pantoprazole 40 mg once a day (coats stomach)
- Dexamethasone 7:00 am and 1:00 pm (steroid)
- Morphine Sulf 5 mg (1-2 every four hours as needed)
- Morphine Sulf Sr. 30 mg 9:00 am and 9:00 pm
- Zinc Vitamin 25 mg 2x day (for bed sores)
- Zopiclone 7.5 mg before bed (for sleep)
- Senokot (to keep things moving)

To make things just a little easier, I got stickers and labelled the lids with what the med was and what it was for. This way when I opened the vanity drawer in our room, away from others, I could tell what each was.

Think about it

Keep a notebook handy. This is super helpful when paramedics come and they need a list of medications. Also, if the doctor wants to know what their vitals were over the past week, the information is at your fingertips.

Inside have...

- A page for doctors' names, phone numbers, and addresses
- A page of medications. (Names and dosages)
- The dates on the top of the remaining pages. (Like an organizer)
- Record vitals on the date page for each day
- Appointments
- Questions for the doctor or nurse, leaving room for the answers
- Notes you take during appointments
- Any changes to medication

On January 11, we went back to St. Marys hospital for Jim to have an ultrasound of his legs because of the swelling. They wanted to rule out blood clots, hoping it was just water gain from his IV fluids on the weekend. They had prescribed Lasix 20 mg once a day for his swollen legs and feet, but the swelling seemed to go down once he was walking around at home, and the fluid started moving. That day at St. Marys he also had chest X-rays.

We met our nurse, Andrea, the following afternoon when she came to our house. She was a sweet young lady who took the time to get to know us and discuss palliative care for us in our situation.

"Doctor Thornton thought it would be a good idea if you came, but I don't know why you need to be here. I'm fine," Jim stated. "I'm much better than I was last week." Looking down in the little brown notebook, I saw a trend showing he had less pain during the day.

"Well, Jim, I'm glad you are letting us come as it does make our job easier. If you are feeling good now, we can keep you this way. If you wait until you are in pain, it is harder for us to get you in a good place," she informed him.

"I guess. I just hate bothering people."

"Well, we will call you every week before coming out. If you feel like everything is good, then we can just chat over the phone," she assured him.

"That sounds like a plan," he said as she took his vitals.

Think about it.

Palliative Care is care to improve the quality of life of patients with serious and life-threatening diseases, such as cancer. It is best to be in palliative care as early as possible so that the symptoms and side effects of the disease and its treatment may be kept under control. It is possible to receive care and then later not need palliative care anymore. But palliative care is the best way to keep patients comfortable on their cancer journey.

Making Plans

THE NEXT DAY, Jessica, Jim's care coordinator through Home and Community Care Support Services, came to the house. She explained that she would be overseeing all the services Jim needed and serving as the main contact person. We would talk to her if we had any issues or concerns and we would likely see her on occasion when the other nurses were on holiday or overloaded with clients. We would also sometimes see Kate, as she was the palliative liaison nurse who sometimes filled in. Jessica filled out a flowchart with all the various names and phone numbers that we might need.

We asked Jessica about the swelling in Jim's legs. She informed us that it had just been water, not blood clots, and he didn't need to take the water pills. She also didn't know why he had a bruise beside his belly button.

Jim also asked about the number of meds he was on. Never having been one for medications, this was a struggle for him to wrap his head around, but after multiple chats, he seemed to understand why he needed them.

"Jim, when you're in pain you're grumpy." I said. "Do you want that to be what your kids remember? I sure don't."

But even this didn't stop him from asking questions.

"Do I have to take the stomach-coating meds twice a day or can I just take one a day with the steroids?"

Yes, he needed it twice a day.

The nurses also arranged for an occupational therapist to assess our house and determine what changes we would need to make so that Jim could stay home as long as possible. They suggested we get a special air mattress for the bed. It would distribute the pressure points and prevent him from getting bed sores.

The occupational therapist then sat down in his recliner, doing a little bounce.

"Since he spends so much time here, you'll need a special air cushion for the chair," she said as she stood up.

She then asked to see the bathroom. Jim followed behind as I directed her around the corner to our larger bathroom. We listened as she suggested we get shower bars to help Jim get in and out of the bathtub.

"I'm not a bath kind of guy," Jim interrupted. "I preferred the shower in the other bathroom." So off we went through the kitchen and down the short hall to the other bathroom. She noted this bathroom didn't have anywhere for Jim to sit while I helped him dress and there was nothing for him to hold on to. She suggested a shower stool, which I knew I could borrow from my mom; she still had my grandmother's.

That night I messaged the kids and explained the needed renovations. I told them what we were thinking, and our two construction sons got their thinking caps on and started texting back and forth, with the other kids contributing a few thoughts of their own. After a day or two, we decided that I would get a quote for installing a wheelchair shower in the big bathroom and removing the clawfoot bathtub, for now.

Jim was realizing how quickly he got winded, but this didn't deter him from visiting his two youngest daughters, Elly and Melissa, who slept upstairs in a large, shared room. Slowly, very slowly, he would pull himself up the stairs. Once at the top, he'd sit and catch his breath in the office chair by the big oak desk he treasured. Finally, he would get up and walk the thirty feet to Elly's bed and sit again, refilling his lungs. He enjoyed being there with the girls while they quietly studied. Other times they would joke and reminisce. He knew they enjoyed this as much as he did. Later, after making several of these trips, Jim found a chair on the landing halfway up the stairs.

One night, Stan, our church elder and a friend of Jim's, came by with his wife. I noticed lately that Jim was extremely talkative when people came to visit. Sure, he was a salesman and could talk, but this was different. He seemed to feel like he had to share everything on his heart at once. Usually I was the talker, but I couldn't get a word in. I reminded myself that the visitors were here for him, not me. I would just let him talk... and talk.

At some point during the visit Jim would declare, "I have had fifty-four great years. God has blessed me more than I could have imagined. I have no regrets." Then, looking at me with tears in his eyes, he would say, "I just wish I could be here when Joanne goes through something like this. I hate the thought of her doing this alone. I could never have done it without her." It was during these visits with dear friends that he would share his feelings with tears in his eyes. Maybe that is why I just let him talk, so I could learn more about how he felt. Even though it was hard to watch him struggle through those words, knowing he was thinking about that meant the world to me. It seemed like each day we were saying less and less to each other.

We each didn't want to upset the other person. We were struggling, knowing that our relationship was coming to an end. We tried to live in the present, but we felt numb. And we tried to ignore the future.

On the evening of January 14, we were blessed when Dr. Thornton came to the house—mask and all. We were surprised to learn that doctors still make house calls. We told her that the Symptom Response Kit had arrived that day. Then she went through the questions we had about a naturopath and supplements. She agreed to send a referral for us to talk with the dietitian at the clinic.

We talked about how much fluid Jim had been getting since Melissa bought him a new water cup with a straw. With his last cup water would spill on the bed because he would fall asleep holding it in his hand. He would joke in the mornings that he just couldn't get to the bathroom in time. Jim was always able to make fun of himself. But the new straw cup was not the greatest for me. Jim would take the straw out of his mouth while still sucking, and the straw would fling water at my face as I lay sleeping. I'd wake up and Jim would quietly say sorry, with a giggle.

The doctor agreed that he was probably dehydrating again, so she ordered an IV. She said there was no hurry; she just wanted to stay on top of it. She let the nurses know they were to put it in for him. She also sent a requisition for an IV pole and fluids to be sent to the house.

Think about it.

A Symptom Response Kit (SRK) includes enough medications and medical supplies to manage the palliative care client's distressing symptoms in the home for up to seventy-two hours. Sometimes referred to as a mini pharmacy in a box, a SRK contains medications to treat common end-of-life symptoms. This kit can help keep the patient at home for treatment instead of taking an ambulance ride while in distress. It helps keep family members more at ease, knowing that help is so close.

The next day, another new nurse came to the house. She tried to connect the IV to give him the fluids that had been delivered to our house. After three unsuccessful tries with the supplies that were found in his System Responds Kit, we agreed to try again tomorrow. We promised to wrap his arm up in warm towels with a hot water bottle an hour before she came, to help bring the veins to the surface.

Meanwhile, Desiree, her husband, and three children arrived early afternoon after a week in isolation. They stayed long enough to give Papa hugs and play with the toys for a short time before her husband, Joey, took the kids down the street to Derek's house to visit their cousins. That evening Joey drove himself and the kids back home to Niagara, where his sister and mom would help him care for the kids. Desiree remained to visit with us for the week.

Then it happened. While cooking dinner, my oven decided to throw a cool light display as its final hoorah. The stovetop worked, just not the oven. While I was a little put out by this, I thought about how upset I would have been if it had happened last year or earlier. I had a different perspective now; A broken oven no longer caused devastating or frustrating thoughts.

Life goes on, and you will continue to have decisions to make in those mundane, daily situations, but there are also more difficult decisions to make. One day I convinced Jim to talk about funeral arrangements, since three of the girls and two boys were in the house. I thought if Jim and I talked with the kids, maybe, just maybe, it wouldn't be so hard. The kids would be the ones going through it, not Jim. Jim agreed reluctantly, and the discussion went well. One of the girls mentioned another funeral we had taken her to.

"I thought it was awful how everyone was at the cemetery gawking at the mourning family. I don't want people there. It should just be for the family." With that in mind, the others leaned toward her train of thought. We decided that on the first day we would have a viewing with the family at the church at 1:00 pm. The casket would then be closed for public visitation from 2:00–4:00 and 7:00–9:00. The next day we would have the funeral in the morning at the church, followed by a luncheon organized by the funeral committee. The interment would be later in the afternoon with only immediate family present. When we had nailed out all the details, we sent them to the other children. I sighed a sigh of relief, knowing these decisions were behind us now.

By this time, we had settled back into a bit of a routine. After getting up in the morning, I would make breakfast while Jim sat drinking his coffee. We would eat breakfast, and then read our devotions together. We were going through a devotional friends had given us, *Truth for Life* by Alistair Begg.[7] Jim and I were so thankful for this book. At the end of each devotion, there were thought provoking questions for us to discuss and relate to our lives. One morning, the Bible reading was from 2 Corinthians 4. Jim

---

[7] Alistair Begg, *Truth for Life: 365 Daily Devotions* (Surrey, England: The Good Book Company, 2021).

was especially excited about verses 16–18: *"Therefore we do not lose heart. Though outwardly we are wasting away, yet inwardly we are being renewed day by day. For our light and momentary troubles are achieving for us an eternal glory that far outweighs them all. So we fix our eyes not on what is seen, but on what is unseen. For what is seen is temporary, but what is unseen is eternal."*

"I have to memorize this one," he said excitedly. So I took a minute to write it out on a recipe card and handed it to him. After reading it over a few times, he placed it on the table beside his chair, where he could read it over numerous times each day.

Following morning devotions, he would shower. I would help him get dressed, as he could no longer bend over. In the past he would have then gone out to feed the chickens, but since being in the hospital, he had only seen them on the camera. Today, he again asked Joshua to feed the chickens and gave instructions from his chair, making sure it was done right.

While listening to the sermon online that morning, we had Jim sitting with his arm wrapped up warm so his veins would be ready for the nurse when she came after the service. He was pretty happy that she was able to get the IV in on the first try.

On Monday morning, the girls let me go grocery shopping and they kept an eye on Dad, who was still attached to his IV pole. After double-checking with them to make sure this was okay, they eagerly encouraged me to go.

"We will just sit here and play Rummikub while you are gone. Maybe some Ninety-Nine too," they said. Ninety-Nine was dad's favourite game and he rarely lost. I grabbed a mask and my grocery bags and headed out the door, leaving him in good hands... or so I thought.

When I arrived home a few hours later, I noticed three people bundled up and walking back from the chicken condo to the house. My mind raced as I panicked and my motherly instincts kicking in. I recognized Desiree and Melissa's snowsuits flanking Jim's. What was he doing outside in the cold? He didn't have the energy to walk that far. Where was his IV? *What were they thinking*? As I got out of the car, they came up to me laughing, a sign they were having a great time.

"What are you guys doing?" I asked as the girls sobered to the familiar *you're-in-trouble* tone.

Jim, still smiling, boldly said, "What bee got in your bonnet?"

I looked him straight in the eye, ignoring the girls who stepped back from his sides. "What did you do with your IV? You were supposed to have it on till it was empty," I said, frustrated.

"I still have it on," he smiled at me. The girls couldn't help but chuckle as he patted his chest.

"What do you mean?" I asked. I was taken aback as he reached to unzip his coat, exposing the IV bag hanging from a lanyard around his neck. Seeing the disbelief on my face, they all burst out laughing as I turned around and quietly went to empty the car of groceries.

That afternoon, the two of us sat side by side on the loveseat in front of the laptop on the coffee table. We had set up a video call with Jeff Lockhart from Lockhart Funeral Home in Mitchell. Unaware of Jim's condition, Jeff, an amiable gentleman, walked us through the different options for preplanning a funeral. He began by asking us what our thoughts and plans were. We explained to him the plans we had made earlier with the kids, and he explained the role of the funeral home in great detail. After we discussed our choice of a cemetery, he suggested we speak to Ben Shackleton from Stratford Memorials about a memorial for Jim.

Now that he knew what cemetery we were looking at, he explained that they each had different rules. Our choice to use Avonbank meant that we couldn't have a burial from November until April. The body would be brought to a mausoleum until after April. He also told us that the cemeteries strongly recommend a concrete vault, but it is not required by law. Jeff then took his iPad and gave us a virtual tour of the casket selection upstairs. This was almost like being there in person. It was interesting to see so many different ones with different details. He then mentioned that we could prepay for a funeral if we would like to. Since we knew we would need his services sooner than later, we decided it would be better to wait for the life insurance money to pay for it. He also encouraged us to look through his website for more information.

Jeff continued discussing the disbursements. These included the cost of the newspaper obituaries and deciding which newspapers we wanted the obituaries to be in. Disbursements also included honorariums for the minister, organist, caretaker, and sound technician, as well as those responsible for the projection and live streaming at the church. He asked us if we wanted a luncheon. I informed him that our church's funeral committee would take care of the luncheon. As for the grave opening cost, he suggested that we pay when we buy our plots. Otherwise, they would put that in the funeral disbursement. Lastly, there was the possibility of a mausoleum fee if someone passed in the winter.

We continued working through a brief outline of the fine details, such as the funeral cards, slide show, register book, and thank you cards. As we discussed the obituaries, Jeff asked if we could email him a list of the names of family members he would need to include. This way he would have all the correct spellings on file. He also needed to know where our parents were born. So, after we had ended our Zoom call with Jeff, I started typing out all the kids' (and spouses) and grandkids' names, along with the names of both Jim's and my siblings (and spouses) and our parents. A few days later, I brought this completed list to their office.

Think about it

Did you know that you can make arrangements at the funeral home of your choice without prepayment? Having arrangements made in advance makes it easier on your loved ones, as they will not need to make hard decisions amid the fog of grief.

A representative from the funeral home will also let you know that the best thing you can do to help the funeral run smoothly is to have a will. A will clearly states who the executor is, which in turn helps the funeral home know who to deal with. Another helpful item is a list of your family members' names, double-checking that they are spelled correctly, along with where your parents were born.

Praise the Lord

THE NEXT DAY we headed back to London for our first meeting with Dr. Logan, the drug (chemo) therapy doctor. Dr. Lang, our radiation doctor, thought it was a good idea to move our appointment earlier. She was concerned about Jim's pain from radiation. In the meantime, Dr. Thornton, our palliative care doctor, had managed to get Jim's pain down to a zero. When Jim did have pain, it was because he was feeling good and doing more than he really should have been. For example, after our neighbour blew out the driveway with the snowblower, Jim went over it again very *slowly* with the snow shovel, taking multiple breaks. But he was able to overcome this pain, which was only at a three out of ten, with a break in his chair instead of more pain meds.

Moving very slowly, we made our way through the clinic to the appointment rooms on the second level, resting when needed. After getting Jim comfortable in a chair, I went to sign him in. We sat there for a while observing those around us, looking at our phones, and discussing again that he didn't want chemo. We had heard that chemo was hard on your body and made you really sick. He didn't want to be sick. He wanted to live out his days as healthy as possible and at home with his family. We had our plan of attack if Dr. Logan was going to say that he wouldn't feel good from chemo.

Jim was finally called in to have his vitals taken. Handing me his winter jacket, he stood on the scale as the nurse had instructed. Saying his weight out loud, Jim was visibly shocked; he had lost over ten pounds in the past week.

"Did you lose a lot of weight?" the observant nurse asked him.

"A lot! My exercise program is working!" His witty humour returned in a flash. She then led us to an unusually large exam room. Again, we waited and waited. Jim talked about just wanting to leave because he was uncomfortable and needed a nap. At one point, I snuck out of the room and inquired about the doctor's whereabouts. They

118

apologized and said she was running behind and would be with us shortly. When Dr. Logan and her resident finally walked in, I looked up at the clock on the other side of the room. Two hours had passed since our arrival. I hoped this wouldn't take long as I also was tired and still had to drive an hour to get home. But I soon forgot about this as this confident, red-headed doctor engaged us with her humour, much like Jim's. Watching Dr. Logan and Jim discussing a serious situation with humour was fun. She clarified that with any treatment or medication, they have an "average" dose that fits ninety-five percent of people. Two percent of people will need more than the average. The remaining three percent of people will need less of the dose. She believed that Jim's radiation from twelve treatments was the same as the "average" others would get with fifteen. Hearing this, we both sighed in relief. We were okay with not having to do the last three treatments.

She told us that Jim looked good and she thought the radiation had accomplished what it what supposed to. But she wouldn't be sure until she saw the results from the CT scan. As for now, she didn't want to give Jim any drugs since he was experiencing next to no pain. This shocked us both. What chemo doctor does not want to give you drugs? She then made sure that we understood that the outcome would still be the same no matter what she did or what the radiation accomplished.

"The purpose of drug therapy, in your case, is to get rid of any annoying symptoms," she explained. Her goal was to help Jim manage the pain, and to be comfortable during the time he had left. The drugs she would give him could make him more tired or cause other side effects. He might be willing to accept those side effects later, in exchange for no pain. But for now she wanted Jim to live life.

That night, after heating a frozen Delissio pizza for dinner, Jim excitedly read Psalm 150, "Let All Things Praise the Lord," for family devotions around the dinner table.

> Praise the Lord.
> Praise God in his sanctuary;
>   praise him in his mighty heavens.
> Praise him for his acts of power;
>   praise him for his surpassing greatness.
> Praise him with the sounding of the trumpet,
>   praise him with the harp and lyre,
>   praise him with tambourine and dancing,
>   praise him with the strings and flute,
>   praise him with the clash of cymbals,

praise him with resounding cymbals,
Let everything that has breath praise the Lord.
Praise the Lord.

Closing the bible, with a huge smile on his face, he again said, "Praise the Lord!" His excitement was contagious. A part of me wanted to share his exuberance, but another part of me wondered if he understood the severity of it all. I didn't want to pull him down; I wanted to take every small victory as a big victory, which is what he was doing. So I echoed him, "Praise the Lord!"

As we felt prayers go up for us, the Lord also opened our eyes to see those struggling around us. That night, as was our custom, we prayed for all our children and for our church family, as well as friends who we knew were struggling. As Jim was staying home and not working, he spent more time thinking about this than I did, I admit. He wanted to be used by God to do more. We agreed that once a week we would write notes to people who we felt needed to know they were being prayed for. We knew how much it meant, having received more than one such note ourselves.

Think about it

When you feel down, is it because you are looking at yourself? What if you looked out, away from yourself, toward others? Try doing something for someone else. Even if it is a little thing, it will make an impact on the other person's life as well as your own. Try it!
"Do nothing out of selfish ambition or vain conceit, but in humility consider others better than yourselves. Each of you should look not only to your own interests, but also to the interests of others" (Philippians 2:3).
"Each helps the other and says to his brother, 'Be strong!'" (Isaiah 41:6).

The next day, Jim mentioned his favourite childhood book, *The Sissy Kid Brother* by Amelia Muiller.[8] We had lent it to someone and never got it back. I had inquired

---

[8] Amelia Mueller, *Sissy Kid Brother* (Pennsylvania, Herald Press, 1975).

if anyone had our copy or maybe had a copy we could borrow, but to no avail. So, what did we do? We ordered it online. Victoria was home that day, so I asked her to purchase it for me.

As it appeared on the screen, her eyes popped, "Mom, it will cost $92.47 with shipping!"

"I know, but he wants it so bad, and he has not asked for anything else," I sighed. I wanted to give him a special gift.

"He wants a new motorcycle!" she laughed.

"Yeah, the book is cheaper when you look at it that way. Just order it." She cringed as her finger hit send, as did I, hoping I made the right choice.

Later that day, feeling helpless, I knew I needed to talk to someone who understood what I was going through. I called my friend Joanne who had lost her husband to a brain tumour ten years earlier. We talked for a bit, I cried, and she understood.

"Just don't forget to tell him you love him," she encouraged. "A lot!" As time progressed, I saw the wisdom in this encouragement.

We had a video call with the dietician from the clinic the following day. Jim explained that he would like to eat in a way that would help him to have more energy and be less tired. She said he needed at least fifteen grams of protein at each meal. He was excited about the prospect of steak! She made other suggestions like cottage cheese, which is high in protein, with berries or other fruit, or with cinnamon and vanilla. We knew more fruits and veggies would also be on the list. She added plain Greek yogurt, salmon, trout, and sardines.

"Sardines! I have not had that since I was a kid! I remember my Dad always eating them." Turning to me, he asked, "Can you get sardines?" I agreed and we listened as she went on to say that dairy products would give him much-needed calcium and vitamin D. Jim also asked if she had heard about sugar causing cancer. She said she had, but only certain types of cancers, and not the type that Jim had.

Once the meeting was over, I bit the bullet and called a family from church who had offered us some beef the week before. I asked if we could get some steaks and roast to help get Jim's iron up. She was so happy I called and was more than willing to drop the meat off that afternoon.

Why was I again surprised at how God works for our good? I had to stomp my pride down and accept the help that was graciously offered to us. This was so hard for me, even though I could see how accepting these blessings was a gift not only for us, but also for those offering the help.

Choices to Make

LATER THAT AFTERNOON, we had a video call with our friend Val who worked at the new hospice in Stratford. The subject of hospice care had been a point of controversy between me and Jim. Jim kept stressing that he did not want to go to hospice *or* the hospital to die. He wanted to stay home with his family around him. I understood and wanted that for him. But what if it would be too hard for the kids to watch him at home? I would be left to deal with post-traumatic stress syndrome too. We didn't know what the end of life would look like. I just wanted to be well-informed. Finally, he agreed to listen to what Val had to say.

After some time catching up, Val explained what hospice care was like. She explained that they make you comfortable in a home-like environment. We asked her about visitors during these COVID times, and she said they were currently only allowing five family members to visit.

"Well, that's it then. I'm not going," Jim stated.

"Yes, that won't work for us, as we don't want to deny any of the kids visiting him," I agreed. Val understood what we were saying and even agreed. She told us that the palliative care teams were really good and would do a good job keeping Jim comfortable. Val then asked Jim if he liked to write. Seeing Jim was a little confused, she explained that before her husband passed away, he had written in a book called *A Father's Legacy*. She explained that it is a book that asks questions about your life and leaves room for you to write the answers below in the book. In the end, you have a story about your life. I thought it would be a great idea. She said her kids loved the book as they can now look back and read about their dad's life in his own handwriting. Jim didn't seem to understand what she was talking about.

She smiled and said, "Jim, I have a copy here. I will drop it off tomorrow and you can look at it and see if that is what you want to do." The next day, as if this conversation had never happened, Jim said he wanted to write about his life for the kids. I had to roll my eyes and laugh. Once he saw the book, he was excited to get started. It had questions about his childhood, family life, education, and jobs. Other questions were about love and marriage, parenting, celebrations, and life events. As he worked through it, though, he found that the space provided was not enough for the stories he wanted to share. He decided that once he finished the book, he would write out the stories on lined paper and staple them to the corresponding pages.

Think about it

Did you know that Hospice care is available in most communities? Lots of care might be needed at the end of life. This care is available in hospice. Take time to discuss with your family where you would like to spend your last days. Hospice care is not only for those at the end of life, it also provides support for their families. This is all done in a relaxing, home-style environment. It is an option for those who don't want to be in the hospital. Maybe you don't want your last days to be at home. Hospice care might be a good option.

Dr. Thornton called that evening. We discussed Jim's fatigue, and wondered if his iron or hemoglobin levels were low. She would order a requisition for tomorrow to get his bloodwork done. Jim had been taking a small dosage of bisoprolol for his high blood pressure, but his blood pressure had improved. She agreed to take him off the bisoprolol. Feeling like he was on a roll, Jim also asked about going off the steroid Dex (dexamethasone).

"I just feel like, no, I *know*, I am short-tempered with the kids. I have no patience with them at all. They don't even want to be around me. I just feel I am agitated all the time," he confessed.

"Yes, that would probably be from the Dex. The only way we'll know is to get you off it. But you can't stop cold turkey, so we can lower your afternoon dose from 4 mg to 2 mg for five days. Are you okay to try that?" Jim agreed, excitedly.

The next day he cut down on his Dex and went for his blood work. Dr. Thornton called again the following day to let us know that his white blood count was way down. She said this was to be expected. Again, she stressed that Jim just couldn't get sick.

That Sunday, after watching church online, Jim announced, "Who is coming for a walk with me down to the river?" to which the kids groaned. "Well, I can't go far or fast, so it won't be too bad. Come on, guys!" Slowly everyone agreed, and we bundled up against the cold air, thankful for the sun shining brightly in the clear blue sky. Walking slowly, we made our way down to the river behind the kids. The lively chatter and fresh air seemed to invigorate him as we got down to the river. Melissa took some photos of us all bundled up and smiling. Ready to turn back, we were all surprised when Jim said he wanted to go farther.

"You do realize you have to walk back, right?" I joked.

"Ha, ha," he sarcastically responded. "I'm feeling pretty good." So, on we walked, watching as the kids threw snow and played just a little too close to the river. When the kids had had enough, they ran ahead back home to warm up while Jim and I sauntered back. We enjoyed the time together, reminiscing about another cold December night when he proposed to me at Niagara Falls.

"You looked so cute in that miniskirt," he said with a smile as his eyebrows hopped up and down.

"Well, it was too cold for that miniskirt. I don't know what I was thinking!"

"I know what I was thinking. *I want to marry this hot young chick!*" We both laughed as we recalled that cold, cold night and how happy we were with the excitement of young love. But the real beauty was that we could remember and be happy without thinking of it as a sad loss.

That next evening Dr. Thornton called again to check on Jim and to ask how weaning off the Dex was going. She decided to keep Jim at the current level. Jim's pain level had increased slightly, and his body was still getting used to the change. Jim also mentioned that his skin felt weird to the touch. It was like he had no feeling in his skin. She found this interesting, but couldn't explain it. This made me sad. He couldn't feel it when I gently held his hand? When I ran my hands down his arms? Anywhere? He was also sad when I talked to him about it.

Taking me in his arms, he squeezed me tight and said, "But I can feel your hugs. I need lots of hugs." We struggled with this new loss.

His nurse Andrea came to the house two days later. Even she noticed how much Jim had perked up and was shocked to see all the little projects he was doing around the house. It was slow going, but he felt useful, he told her. Noting this in my mind, I knew I had to let him putter no matter how much I wanted him to rest. This is what he needs to do right now. As the appointment came to a close, Jim told her he didn't think he needed palliative care. He felt like a bother when others were in worse shape than him. They agreed that she would call once a week to check on him and see if he felt he needed a visit.

In the past, I had known of only one person that Jim struggled with. He felt he was ill-treated by this person when he was a child. Jim mentioned that he wanted to find this person and talk to them, hoping to figure out the past. But deep down, I knew he wanted this person to ask him for forgiveness. He wanted to know if they thought about him and the situation as he did.

I suggested looking up the person on Facebook. We did and found them. Since Jim didn't have Facebook, he used mine and sent a long, polite message. He said nothing of the past, only a friendly hello and some info to catch them up on the time that had gone by. He was excited to receive a lengthy message back, with a warm greeting and news of what had happened in this person's life since they last met. Jim was disappointed that nothing was said about the issue all those years ago.

"Honey, you were a kid then. Is it possible that it got bigger in your mind over the years than theirs?" I tried to say this gently, realizing it was probably not the right thing to say as the sparks flew from his eyes. I decided to try another approach. I crouched down in front of him and reached for his hands as he sat in his chair. "Hon, you reached out. You gave them the opportunity. They know your situation. Now it is *you* who has to forgive and let it go," I said tenderly. He was thinking while looking down at our hands in his lap. I could see the wheels turning as he tried to forgive and forget.

"It's hard. It has been so long I have carried it around," he said, looking up at me with sad eyes. Telling him I loved him and squeezing his hands, I left him and prayed silently that he would be able to let it go. As I looked back, I could see him fold his hands and lay his head back, closing his eyes.

Think about it

Jesus has shown what real love, mercy, and forgiveness look like by dying on the cross for our sins. If you follow Him, then you should forgive those around you. Maybe that's a co-worker or someone you knew a long time ago like a past teacher or an old friend who hurt you in some way. It might be someone closer like your parents or a sibling. But you have to let it go before it is too late. Will you extend love, mercy, and forgiveness? Forgiving someone might be hard, but isn't it worth all of eternity?

"'Shouldn't you have had mercy on your fellow servant just as I had on you?' In anger his master turned him over to the jailers to be tortured, until he should pay back all he owed. 'This is how my heavenly Father will treat each of you unless you forgive your brother from your heart'" (Matthew 18:33–35).

Thursdays were exciting for Jim. His dear friend Tim Van de Kemp would stop by to encourage him in between stops on his dry-cleaning delivery route. Jim highly respected and looked up to Tim as a fellow homeschooling dad and elder in the church. He was one of the people Jim would go to for advice. This week Tim brought over a book he had just written called, "A New Life in a New Land." The book is about Tim's family's immigration to Canada in May of 1954. Jim was eager to read it as his sales area used to be around Atwood when he worked for Listowel Premiere, the same area where Tim's family had first arrived by train. Jim loved history books, so it wasn't surprising when he spent all day and night reading Tim's book. I'm not kidding, day and night! I would wake up in the night to Jim reading, with his side of the bed up and his phone light on. Groaning, I would roll over, away from the light reflecting off the page, hoping he would read faster.

On Friday we had a social worker call us from the home care coordinators. She would help with any paperwork Jim needed to complete, including the Disability Tax Credit and Critical Illness Insurance that the doctor suggested we look into. She promised she would look into these things more and get back to us.

Sundays were getting harder as words to each song seemed to hit us in some way. This particular Sunday, the words to the song "He Knows My Name" by Tommy Walker[9] made his eyes glisten. We knew God was working in us, as we didn't feel anger toward Him. We knew He had a plan that was bigger than us, one we couldn't see. But as the song lyrics said, He would never leave us no matter where we went. Resting in that assurance, we continued to trudge on.

---

[9] Tommy Walker, "He Knows My Name," Doulos Publishing (BMI), 1996.

A Secret, Lost

THROUGH IT ALL, we tried to find ways to enjoy life and make new memories. When Jim's mom had asked me a few weeks earlier what I wanted for my birthday, my answer was, "Time with your son." She made it possible for us to head off to Benmiller Inn and Spa in Goderich that sunny day, January 31. The kids were concerned. To keep him safe, they hadn't been allowed to visit Dad. But now we were going out in public.

But we needed time out of the house—time with just the two of us, having received the dreadful news only six weeks earlier. When we arrived, I went in to register and found out we were the only guests. This was their off-season and they had just reopened due to COVID. I took great joy in letting the kids know their dad was safe.

It was a beautiful multi-levelled room with all the perks. The far wall of windows would be beautiful when the sun rose over the river and a field beyond as we lounged in bed the next morning. But for now, we sat side by side on the couch and talked. I had taken twenty conversation starter questions all typed up and cut into little strips in a small Tupperware container. I explained to him that since this was my birthday trip, I wanted to go through these questions. When he started rolling his eyes at me I reassured him that I wouldn't make him do it all in one sitting, and I promised it would be fun. Some required short answers that didn't take much thought, but others required longer answers. For those longer ones we took time to think before writing out our answers on paper. Once done, we exchanged papers and read each other's answers.

One of the long questions was, "If you could have lunch with anyone in the world, who would it be and why?" I was slightly surprised by Jim's answer, "I think right now, because I read his book and he is someone I have always admired and respected, it would have to be Tim van de Kemp. Yes, that's it!" But the more I thought about it, the more I could see why that was his answer.

Another question was, "List three things you would like to do before the next year passes." Jim's answers didn't surprise me as we had talked about them more often lately.

1. A family gathering with my entire family. Maybe for Easter?
2. A holiday with Joanne where we go out on the motorcycle. Just a holiday together.
3. A family camping trip again with our entire family.

Leave it to Jim to break the rules by adding a fourth answer: Have lunch with Tim.

We also pulled the question, "List three things you would like to do in the next five years." Jim looked at me. "I probably won't be here in five years," he stated matter-of-factly.

"Possibly, but we don't know that, so let's just play along now, shall we?" Shrugging his shoulders, he started to think. "Where is your hope anyway?" I said as an afterthought, trying to get past his observation to the question at hand.

"Oh, I got *hope*, but God has a plan," he said, still looking down at his paper while playing with his pen. I had noticed lately that he was spending more time than usual with the Lord. I could see heaven was heavy on his heart, for him and his family. He was becoming that man I had always dreamed I would marry, leading our family closer to God and encouraging me to lean more on God too. This man beside me now was a different Dad than he was with the older kids. Do they see the change in him?

After spending only a short time, as promised, on a few more questions, Jim encouraged me to go for a walk. This didn't surprise me, as Jim always loved the great outdoors. But as we started walking, I realized that my classy knee-high boots were not made for hiking. Having followed the road a little way to a dead end, he saw a path going off to the right, up the side of a hill. Following his adventurous spirit, he started to follow it.

"Jim, what are you doing?" I said, slightly exasperated.

"Come on, hon, this will be fun! Where is your adventurous spirit?"

"Back at our room in the hot tub!" I declared as I stood at the bottom, watching him struggle up the steep incline using skinny trees to help pull himself up. Sighing deeply, I took the first two steps, sliding back one. Taking two more quick steps, I slid back down to the bottom.

Laughing, I said, "Jim, I don't have the right boots for this!"

"Come on! You can do it. Use the trees." With stomping feet pointing out like a duck, and with the help of the trees, I began the slow, steep incline. Halfway up, I caught up to him while he rested against a tree.

"How are you doing this? I am out of air," I questioned.

"I think I understand now what you always told me about your asthma," he said, trying to catch his breath. Looking up the hill and then back at me, "Are you ready to finish the climb?" Looking down the hill and back at him, "Looks safer than the other option." So, on we went, getting to the top with a little more ease as it levelled out just a little. We followed a trail that forked until we came to a sign that said we were entering Falls Reserve Conservation. Turning back to the fork, we took the other route which led us around to a subdivision. Here we walked for a bit, looking at the different houses, saying what we would or wouldn't like for our house or a future smaller house. Again, we found ourselves comfortably talking about our dreams like it was a normal thing to talk about. Which it was, but maybe not for us.

Later that evening, we laughed at the number of extra pillows they had put in our room. I had asked for extra to ensure Jim would have a good sleep. Getting comfy in each other's arms surrounded by fluffy pillows, we talked about more intimate things. Holding me close, Jim apologized that he couldn't show me how much he loved me. The look in his eyes made my heart break in two. I could see he felt like a failure. He didn't know what to do. He tried to say it in words but knew that it wasn't the same. We cried together. We cried over the loss of yet another thing in our lives, the loss of a healthy physical relationship. I was past the disappointment of the past months; now, I was just angry. I was not ready to let that chapter in our lives go. But as we lay there, I acknowledged the conflicting emotions raging through my heart, and I didn't feel very holy. I knew I shouldn't be angry. This was not his fault. He was not doing this on purpose. The radiation and the drugs had done this to his body. I had to show him that I loved him, for him, not for the physical act of marriage. I started to hatch a plan in my mind. As I snuggled in closer to him, I asked him if he remembered when we were dating and in love.

"Remember how we used to tease each other with a wink across the room, a flirtatious word or a note? Remember how we would hold hands or just hold each other? Why don't we do that again? Let's just pretend we are dating. We can find happiness in each other that way, can't we?" I asked with hope in my voice.

"Are you sure? It won't be the same."

"Yeah, it's not going to be the same, but we get disappointed every time we force this. Dating again would be different, but at least the disappointment would be gone. The pressure would be off."

After some thought, he asked, "You are sure?" I said I was and we agreed that from now on there would be lots of hugs and flirtations comments even if it grossed out the kids. And believe it or not, it was downright fun!

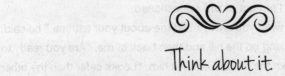

Think about it

Change is something we fear; we become anxious and feel out of control. We have to remember to trust God, for he has a plan. Allowing change can bring us closer to Jesus. Keep changing, finding new ways to live and love.

"Therefore, if anyone is in Christ, he is a new creation; the old has gone, the new has come! All this is from God, who reconciled us to himself through Christ and gave us the ministry of reconciliation" (2 Corinthians 5:17–18).

The next morning, after a surprisingly good sleep for both of us, I went to the washroom. Coming back to bed, I found Jim propped up on one arm, watching me with a smile beaming on his face. Behind him the sun rose, not to disappoint, showing beautiful bright red, orange, and yellow colours trimmed in with purple in an open blue sky. As I drew closer, I noticed a small package from Swanson Jewelers in Stratford on my pillow.

"Happy Birthday! Open it! I had it specially made just for you," he said giddily. I opened it to find a beautiful toonie-sized pendant on a necklace. The pendant had a circular outline containing a tree in the middle. On the tree were ten birthstones to represent all ten of our kids. Together, huddled on the bed, we looked up a birthstone legend on his phone and tried to figure out whose was whose.

"At first, I asked for a charm for your charm bracelet but there were too many stones to make that work," he laughed. "So, Deb suggested I make it into a necklace."

"I love it. I can wear it when I wear my charm bracelet!" I am not a big jewelry person, but I loved this necklace. It had so much meaning. It represented our life with the two of us, working to raise children day in and day out; our children were our life.

After eating breakfast that I had packed for us, we headed out for a leisurely stroll. No more of this mountain climbing stuff. After that, we packed up and headed home, contemplating going out for dinner. Not wanting to take the risk of missing our appointment with Dr. Thornton, we decided to go straight home. At home we shared our mountain climbing adventures with the kids, while laughing at ourselves. Soon after, we were on the call with Dr. Thornton, again discussing reducing the Dex and getting a refill of the morphine.

Burst of Energy

THE FOLLOWING DAY we went to Stratford for another CT scan. We asked if they could have the images sent to Dr. Lang in time for Jim's radiation checkup the next day. They promised to try their best.

We had scheduled a video call for that afternoon with Jan and Wilma in Holland. We told them Jim was feeling much better, and we didn't know for how long. We encouraged them to come soon, if they were serious about coming. We also stressed how important it was that Jim not get sick. Sadly, we also had to let them know we wouldn't be able to go to many places with them when they were here. They understood and would try to get a flight as soon as possible.

We laughed the next day when we received a picture of their plane tickets dated for only three weeks later. They were coming. This was both exciting and scary, as they would be coming by plane through a busy airport. Who knew what they might pick up on their way here? Some of our kids were very concerned about our decision to let them come. We understood this concern well.

The next day Jim drove as we made our way to the cancer clinic. Dr. Lang met with us with good news. "Inside, the tumours look dead. The 24 centimetre tumour is now down to 17 centimetres; there doesn't seem to be any more mets. This is the best possible outcome." She reassured us with a smile. She went on to say that he responded well to the treatments and mentioned that the fast-growing tumours had been alarming to her as well. She reassured us that the twelve treatments were good as they were only aiming for ten treatments. Booking the next CT scan for April, the plan was to watch and wait to see what would happen.

Elly and Melissa had been doing their university courses online, from home. The schools were going back to in-person, and they were unsure what they should do. They knew if they left, they wouldn't be allowed back into the house as they could easily pick up illnesses. Finally, Jim said it was their decision and told them not to regret whatever they decided. He said he would love to have them home, but understood that they had to go on with their lives too. We didn't know how long this would be, and he was feeling much better right now. After thinking it over, they each decided to make their way back to school. Elly left the first week of February, while Melissa waited a few more weeks.

I had been noticing changes in Jim for a while. I asked my older kids if they had also noticed these changes. Some of them said Dad was still his goofy old self. Finally, on February 4, I sent a message to Dr. Thornton, "I need to tell you, without Jim knowing because I don't want to worry him, his mannerisms are changing. Some days I also wonder if something is happening in his brain. He has less patience. He forgets things and sometimes mixes up information. They are not huge things, but I notice them and think a few others have too. He talks more than he ever has before. In the past, if I asked a question, he would take his time to answer. Now he tries to answer before I even finish the question. I do not know if this is connected to the loss of sensation that he is having. I decided to pass on this information after my son asked me if necrosis was an issue. I had never heard of it before. When I googled necrosis, I read, 'Necrosis can occur due to injuries, infections, or diseases. Lack of blood flow to your tissues and extreme environmental conditions can cause necrosis. While dead body tissue can be removed, it can't be brought back to good health.'"

Doctor Thornton soon replied, "Thanks, this sounds like hypomania from the dex." She promised to review his tapering schedule and arrange the fastest way to get him off. She would suggest a CT of his head if he didn't respond. Without anyone knowing any of this, I began to pray that he would be able to get off the dex, and that this would improve the situation. I knew he was frustrated with himself for being short with the kids. I wanted these end days to bring good memories for everyone.

Meanwhile, at home, Jim found a burst of energy and took it upon himself to fix the crown moulding in the dining room. Sitting in his chair, and looking up at the fourteen-foot ceilings, he declared that he was disgusted at how the trim was never finished properly. He went to the garage and brought in the ladder. Then he sat on his chair for a rest. After a few minutes, he went to the mudroom for the caulking and gun. After another short rest, he slowly made his way to the laundry room for a rag and a pail, stopping at the kitchen to fill up the pail as he sat on an island chair. Once the pail was full, he carried it over to the ladder and climbed up, pail and rag in hand. Reaching the trim, he washed the section he could reach. Climbing back down, he sat on the couch, taking slow, deep breaths. After a few minutes, he went up again, this time with the caulking gun and another rag. Once the seam was filled to his satisfaction, he made his way back down to the couch for another rest. He then began to move the ladder around the room to each seam while taking couch breaks between ladder climbs. It was painstakingly slow to watch, so I kept myself busy in the kitchen, staying nearby in case he needed me. As the day progressed, he was able to make two trips before resting. By the evening he didn't want to rest; he was on a roll. I forced him to go to bed, only to watch him start slowly again the next day, gaining energy as the day went on.

After the caulking was done, Jim decided the trim needed a coat of paint. Once this was done, he announced that the huge windows needed painting to match the fresh white trim. At one point during the window trim painting, his friend Rene from Alberta—who was best man at our wedding—texted him to see how he was. He would get up the ladder to the window to paint, and a text would appear on his phone below. Climbing down, he would answer the text. After climbing up again, another text would come in. After doing this for a while, I told him just to sit and have a conversation. Instead, he took the phone up with him so he could paint and text.

These windows are attached to the wainscoting that goes around half of this large room. While painting the wainscoting, he came to the doorways. On one door frame we have recorded all our children's heights over the past nineteen years. With ten children, there is lots of writing on this frame! The FamJam was abuzz about what we should do with the frame. Some suggested we "cover it." Others suggested we "take it out and replace it so you can keep it." In the end, we decided to leave it, and I traced the faded writing to make it stand out

On Tuesday, Jim drove us to Stratford Memorials for our appointment with Ben Shackleton. Ben asked us where we considered being buried, as each cemetery has its own rules. We smiled at each other as we told him Avonbank. He let us know that the price of the stone included the design on the front and the back. We could get a picture or words on the stone, whatever we wanted. Jim saw one with a picture of a farm which got him thinking how nice that would be. Quietly disagreeing, we agreed we would talk more about it later. Ben took us outside to see the different stones. There were different sizes, shapes, and colours. We effortlessly agreed on a basic black one. With the stone agreed upon, we got a ballpark figure from Ben before we left. We tried to hold our jaws up at the big number. But what were we to do? Also, due to COVID, the stones were taking longer to come in. It would be four to six months before it would be completed. He promised to send an email with the quote by the next day.

We discussed what we would put on the stone as we drove home. Jim felt that his love for farming should be represented on the stone with a farm scene. I reminded him it was to be my stone also, and farming was not my thing. Also, we never lived on a life-sustaining farm. I just wanted to include what really mattered to us, our faith.

I wanted a whole text from the Bible written out so people could read it. I didn't just want the reference, as no one would look it up. Jim understood what I was saying, and agreed. Before our meeting with Ben, Jim had already found a verse, Psalm 127:4–5: "*Like arrows in the hands of a warrior are sons born in one's youth. Blessed is the man whose quiver is full of them. They will not be put to shame when they contend with their enemies in the gate.*" After reading the entire Psalm that evening, we agreed that we wanted a picture of a quiver with ten arrows. The following night Jim read Psalm 128. He thought that might be an option too.

Pastor Martin came to visit the following afternoon. He was ready to encourage us to talk about funeral plans. To his surprise, Jim told him we had already worked through all that and were in the process of working on the headstone. Pastor Martin said he wasn't aware of another couple who had worked on a stone together before either had passed away. When I thought more about it, I thought about how hard that would be to do by myself right after losing him.

Think about it

You might want to walk through a cemetery to see how different people have designed their memorials. Think about what you want to be remembered for. What special touches would represent your life? Talk with your loved ones about what you would like on your monument. Making a pencil sketch is helpful to file or take with you when you learn more about what styles of memorials are available. (Make sure you write what you want, word for word, so spelling errors can be avoided.) There are many different styles, sizes and colours to choose from. Making these decisions will lessen the load on your grieving family. Once you select your stone, they will help fine-tune your sketch.

Desiree's family came for another visit after being in isolation for a week. They stayed for a longer visit this time as Jim was feeling better than the last time. Before coming, Jim and Desiree had made plans to replace the bathroom countertop. Nathan had made a trip to Home Depot for us. On a video chat he showed me what was available.

After making a decision, he delivered the countertop to our garage and it was ready for Desiree's arrival.

The day arrived and Jim and Desiree took the vanity out. Once it was out, they cut out the hole in the floor where the heat duct was supposed to have gone when the bathroom had been done a handful of years earlier. Figuring where it was to go, Jim took the skill saw and began cutting. From the kitchen, I heard the saw stop.

"Uh-oh!" Jim said as Desiree gasped.

"Don't tell your Mom," he said with a snicker.

"I heard! What did you do?" I asked, not wanting to see the destruction. Then I heard the duct tape being unrolled and slapped down.

"You hear *nu-thing*!" he said only somewhat convincingly.

"He just tried to back the saw up, and it took off through the flooring," Desiree spilled.

"But it's all good. It will be under the vanity, and no one will see it," he said. I'm sure he gave Desiree the "you snitch" look.

The two of them went to the basement to connect the ductwork. Desiree climbed into the crawlspace under the bathroom, looking back to see her dad come in after her.

"I can do this, Dad," she said, still wondering if he was as well as he looked.

"I know you can. I just want to do it with you."

Later, with the ductwork in place, and the vanity hiding the duct-taped floor, they figured out the placement of the sinks on the countertop. After it was all marked out, Jim gave Desiree the okay to start cutting the holes.

"Are you sure? You trust me?" she asked, a little skeptical, not really trusting herself.

"Yep, go for it!" he said enthusiastically.

As she cut, I remembered a story they told me about a father-daughter night at the Gems girls club years ago. The dads and daughters were to pound a nail into a piece of wood as a team. He told me that many watched in astonishment as Jim lightly tapped in the nail to get it started, but left the rest, handing the hammer to Desiree. Proudly he stepped back to watch as she pounded that nail in. Over the years, Jim has taught our kids many useful skills. Who knows when they might come in handy?

Having the counter all cut and in place, they went to work on oil changes and other vehicle maintenance with some of the other kids. Yes, he was frustrated that he couldn't do a simple job as quickly as he would like. But he was still able to do it. Needless to say, he was kept very busy.

"I would have never thought you would be doing this a month ago, Jim!" Dr. Thornton said the following Tuesday. Andrea, the nurse, and I agreed. Our family felt very blessed to have this extra "healthy" time with Jim. We would take every day we had, thankful for each one.

As the older boys suggested, we had someone come out to look at the bathroom. The gentleman thought it would be a pretty straightforward renovation since the bathroom was big and there was lots of room to work with. He gave us a quote after we sat down to pick shower stall panels, faucets, and handrails. Swallowing slowly, we said we would get back to him. After he left, we sent a photo of the quote to the boys. They said, "We could renovate your whole bathroom, not just the shower, for that price!" So back to the drawing board we went.

Jessica, the social worker, encouraged Jim to look at the Assistance Device Program (ADP) to get help with the bathroom renovation. She said the March of Dimes charity might also be able to help with the costs. So off we went to do more investigating.

More Ups and Downs

JIM WAS AGAIN having a hard time isolating himself at home. Being a people person, he needed company to keep his spirits up. On the other hand, was it worth the risk of catching COVID? Finally, he made up his mind that we were going to have company. He just needed company.

"Anyone who wants to come can come," he told me. "I don't want you to turn anyone away. Just make sure they keep their distance and understand that I can't get sick."

"I know this is what you need, but what about the kids?" I asked, feeling stuck in the middle.

"What do you mean, about the kids?" he asked.

"If you get to have friends, the kids will ask why they can't have friends over too."

"Because I can't get sick," he said angrily.

"I am not trying to start an argument. I am letting you know that this is the conversation we will be having with the kids, and we need to be on the same page when we tell them."

After taking a minute to think and calm down, he responded, "Well, maybe we can let them have friends over, but they have to be outside for a walk or something." We told the kids they could have friends over, but they had to do an outside activity while trying to properly distance themselves. With this information out, people started requesting visits. So, together we rearranged the dining room so that Jim and I would sit on one side and guests on the other side.

Two cadet counsellors came with a big card full of notes and signatures from the cadets. We sat and laughed as Jim reminisced about his years involved in this boys' program. It was something he loved.

"I remember my first year as a counsellor. I was sixteen, seventeen. I even took those boys out camping at the Pinery by myself. They would never let you be a counsellor on your own at that age anymore."

He continued, "I remember doing fun stuff with the boys. Then when we would come in from outside or walk through the big room, Dirk would be there shaking his head disapprovingly." He said this with a smile as Dirk sat across from him. "But we were having fun. It was a good time!" Jim shared many cadet stories that day. He had mentored boys in the program since he was a teenager. He continued during our years in Georgetown when we were first married. And later, when the kids were little, this was his thing. It was important to him. For a few years, he was behind the scenes trying his hand at being the head counsellor. But that wasn't where his heart was. He wanted to be in there with the boys, not behind the scenes planning. He did take a few years off when the older boys were finished, but was right back in there when our younger boys were old enough.

One day, I answered a knock on the door to find a neighbour who had heard about Jim and wanted to see him. Jim was not having a good day, so I tried to deter the neighbour, asking him to come another day. When this didn't work, I left him at the door, promising to ask Jim if he was up to a visit. Once in the dining room, I noticed the neighbour had followed behind me, ready for a visit. Jim's eyes flew open as he stood by the wood stove warming up. I could see the panic in his eyes as the neighbour boldly went to shake Jim's hand in greeting. I was able to step between them, explaining that we had to keep our distance to keep him safe. Jim motioned for him to sit on the other side of the room while Jim sat in his recliner. This was a stressful visit; we were on the edge of our seats. Once this well-meaning neighbour left, with a smile and encouraging words on his lips, we breathed a sigh of relief.

My cousin Sherry, who was recovering from yet another sarcoma cancer surgery, explained that her cancer, like Jim's, was a soft tissue cancer. She was a wealth of information, having done a lot of research on cancer, radiation, and chemo treatments. She had chosen only to have surgery, and she explained some of the things she had discovered about radiation that we had already noticed happening to Jim. We discussed how the two of them got this type of cancer. We acknowledged that we all have cancer cells in our bodies that are inactive. In her research, Sherry had found something that suggested that it might come from trauma to that area. She shared the trauma she experienced earlier in life to the cancer area in her body. Jim recalled a time when he was carrying something, not seeing what lay ahead; he walked into a post sticking out of a skid at leg level. He had wondered if that was how his cancer started.

The following Friday, Jim went out to slowly snow blow the driveway. Later that morning, Tim and Betty Van de Kemp were coming to take us on a "book tour." Jim was over-the-moon excited. Once they arrived, Betty and I climbed in the back seat of Jim's pickup, and Tim climbed in the passenger seat with a book and map in hand.

It was a fun day as we drove through the countryside looking at buildings that had been changed into different buildings and seeing places where buildings were no more. Jim shared stories of customers and Tim of his long-ago neighbours. It was a long day for Jim, but a good day that Jim and Tim would treasure.

That night Jim was even more anxious about getting winded so quickly. I encouraged him to call the palliative care nurse, as they kept reminding us to call whenever we needed anything. He finally gave up arguing, 'I don't want to bother them,' and called. After explaining the situation, she encouraged Jim, if he felt okay with it, to wait until his appointment with Dr. Thornton on Tuesday, but if it got any worse, to go to the emergency department.

We woke to a snowstorm the next morning. Having forgot to pick up Jim's refill medication the day before, we had no choice but to brave the snow. On the way, in our four-wheel drive, we saw many vehicles in the ditch. I made a short video of the nearly invisible road and people in the ditch and sent it to Jan and Wilma, saying we looked forward to their visit in four days. Jan said he would be staying home if it was like that. He didn't like the cold. We reassured him we had a nice warm woodstove he could cozy up to.

After taking his meds, Jim bundled up in his insulated overalls, big winter coat, hat, and mitts and headed out to the chicken condo. With the wind and snow whipping around him, he slowly trudged through the path filling in with snow. Once the chickens were fed and watered, he headed back with eggs in his pockets. Halfway back, he found himself without air and scared. He stood still, trying to catch his breath. What was he to do? He couldn't just sit down in the snow. It was too cold, and no one would come. He had to make it back to the house. He forced himself the rest of the way uphill to the other side of the house and into the mudroom. Calvin heard him and ran to the kitchen to get me.

"Dad's in the mudroom. He is making funny noises," he told me with fear in his voice. I ran to Jim and found him leaning over the workbench. He could hardly breathe. I quietly talked to him, encouraging him to breathe. After about five minutes, his breathing started to return to normal. I helped him out of his snow clothes while he did minimal moving. After waiting for more time to pass, we went into the living room, where he sat in the rocking chair for about ten minutes. Then, as I walked next to him for support, he made it to the hall, where he had to stand still to take deep breaths before moving to his chair in the dining room.

By the afternoon, he felt much better. He told me he still had to look for that fourth egg and fix something in the chicken condo. This time I went with him. To make the trip a little easier, we started and ended at the front door, which was closer than the mudroom door. It was slow going, and we took lots of rests along the way.

That afternoon Jim called the nurse, letting her know what had happened earlier that day. After talking with Dr. Thornton, the nurse encouraged us to go to the emergency department. They suspected he might have blood clots in his lungs. CT scans were ordered again, but there were no appointments till the morning. We were sent home for the night with instructions to go to Stratford at 8:00 am then returning to St. Marys emergency department for the results. In the meantime, they put Jim on 10 mg of Apixaban—blood thinners—to fight against blood clots.

While waiting in an old operating room at the back of the St. Marys emergency department, I again realized how this disease was taking its toll on our happiness. We were uncomfortable talking about life, the real life we were living each and every day. I was hesitant to say anything because I didn't want to upset him. Maybe he felt that way too, not wanting to upset the delicate balance we seemed to have found. I think we joked around to hide the fact that we hurt inside for the things we had lost. Therefore we trudged on, all the while knowing there would be more that we would lose.

Jim perched his small phone screen on a little stainless-steel table in the room, and we pulled our two chairs up close to watch the morning church service. Halfway through the sermon, a familiar doctor came in. She introduced herself to Jim. She apologized for the long wait as we got lost in the shuffle for a bit. Then she told us the bad news. Jim had tumours in his lung. We smiled.

"Yes, we know that. We are here to find out if there are any blood clots. The doctor last night was concerned there might be blood clots." Shock followed by relief passed over her face as she looked at us for a minute before looking down at the file in her hand, giving it another quick read.

"No, there does not seem to be. But there might be a pocket of infection. I'm going to put you on some Amoxicillin 875mg with Clavulanate pot for seven days." She explained that the Amox was for the infection and that the pot was to help with the discomfort.

With the script in hand, we left the hospital reflecting on the wasted day, but thankful Jim didn't have to stay. That evening Dr. Thornton called and said Jim should take the medication for ten days just to be safe. We had also noticed a flux in his pulse with these new meds. So, two nights later, Dr. Thornton called again to ask how his pulse was doing. We also discussed lowering the Dex just a little more. He was starting to feel more tired again. I asked her if it might be because his iron was low. She didn't think this was low iron, just the progression of the disease. Jim was determined that he wanted to double-check all his options. I knew we had been over all the options multiple times, but he needed the reassurance that he had done everything he could. I was so thankful for Dr. Thornton's patience with us, as Jim seemed to forget what she said. Dr. Thornton and I would turn to him and gently repeat ourselves like it was the first time he asked. She promised Jim she would contact Dr. Lang, his radiation doctor, to see if any more radiation could be done.

One day, Joshua, our youngest, and I were alone when I broached the topic of Dad. I wanted to know how he was doing with all of it.

"I'm mad!" he stated.

"Mad? Why mad?" I questioned in surprise.

"Dad keeps saying, 'Not bad for an old guy!' when someone asks how he is doing. Well, he is going to *die*! He makes people think he is fine, and then *we* will be left to tell them he died. It will be a shock for all these people," he wisely reasoned. "Why does he do that?"

"I don't know Josh. Maybe you should ask him," I suggested.

"No, that will just get him mad at me," he said quietly. My heart hurt for him.

"Are you okay if I talk to him about it?" I asked.

"Sure, whatever," he said. Later that night, I talked to Jim about it.

"He has a point, dear," I reasoned.

"Yes, but I don't know how to say it well."

"How about something like, 'The cancer is filling my lung, and it doesn't look good. I'm enjoying life while I still can,' and then move on to how they are," I suggested.

"It bothers him that much?" he questioned after thinking a while.

"Yes, it does."

"Well, I guess I have to work on that then," he stated.

Our daughter Elly was lounging on the couch Wednesday morning, talking with Jim, when Dr. Thornton called back. Like always, Jim had her on speaker phone so I could listen in too. She told us that Dr. Lang said that Jim had used up his lifetime use of radiation. If he had any more, it would do more harm than good. Dr. Lang would get in touch with Dr. Fortin, his lung surgeon, so that Jim could talk to her one more time. He knew the answer but just needed to talk to her for his own peace of mind. This left Dr. Logan, the chemo doctor. They would set up a meeting with her to get something started.

"Jim, Dr. Lang and I came up with a timeline. Did you want to know what it is?" she asked him calmly. Jim slowly looked up at me from across the room, thinking.

"No, I don't think so," he said peacefully. I smiled and nodded to him, supporting his decision. She finished by promising to get back to us as soon as she heard back from the other doctors.

As Jim started drafting an email to the minister and our older kids, Elly followed me into the kitchen. "Mom, do you want to know how much time Dad has?" she wondered aloud.

Taking a minute to think, I smiled at her, "I agree with Dad. If we know the time they give him, we will get more sad as it gets closer. But if we don't know the timeline, then we can just enjoy each day as it comes. And you have to remember, Elly, they do not know the time; only God does." I could see she was pondering that as she moved on.

• • •

Today I received word from my medical team regarding my current health status. The nature of the metastasis discovered in my left pleura, along with the multiple rapidly growing nodes, indicates the disease is running rampant and has taken a life of its own. Radiation is no longer considered a viable option. I will still have a discussion with the radiologist, but no radiation is the consensus at this point. I will also be meeting with a doctor to discuss chemotherapy, but have already been told there is no real effective treatment for my condition. (Chemo offers a 30 percent success rate at best.) Also, chemo would greatly decrease my quality of life. I've also asked to meet with the thoracic surgeon, but I know already she will not likely recommend surgery. So, today we are just trying to take this all in. It seems grim, to say the least, but we know there is hope, maybe not in the sense of physical healing, but we have hope just the same. Within the next week or so, we will learn more, but this is what we know so far.

Laughter with Friends

WE WELCOMED JAN and Wilma into our home late that night amid smiles, tears, and hugs. After having pie and tea, my parents, who graciously picked them up for us, said goodnight and began their two-hour drive home.

We visited at home the next morning while we waited for Jim's oxygen machine to arrive. We went through photo albums of our trip to Holland in 2018, laughing at the good times we had. We also went through our wedding albums from thirty-two years earlier, their last visit to Canada. We shared stories and memories and laughed some more. It felt so good to laugh again. Understanding that we couldn't do the touristy things, they graciously said they just wanted to see how and where we lived. They also wanted to meet our children and see their homes. So, we began making arrangements to safely visit the kids. We knew this would be hard as we hadn't seen the grandkids for a while, and the urge to hug them would be great.

Later that morning, two young ladies came and set up Jim's oxygen machine for us. The bottom unit took the air from the room and purified it. The smaller unit on top was a refuelling station so we could fill smaller tanks to take with us when we went out. The white plastic grocery bag was full of yards and yards of clear hose and extra nose prongs.

When we arrived at St. Jacob's Market that afternoon, we were surprised to see very few people. Secretly Jim and I were excited at the prospect of walking around with Jan and Wilma without worrying about being too close to people. After finding a place to park, we bundled up and began walking the outdoor thoroughfare. After about twenty paces, Jim was slowing down considerably. He encouraged Jan and Wilma to walk around, while we found a bench close by.

"Why don't you try the oxygen tank? This would be the perfect time to see if it's helpful or not," I encouraged, not wanting either of us to sit in the cold.

"I guess it's worth a try," he said, slowly getting up. We sauntered back over to the truck. He took off his coat to strap on the tank. I realized he was trying to hide it as he pulled his coat back on, stuffing the extra tube length in and zipping his jacket up higher than before. "There, all set!" he said, grabbing my hand and heading back to where we had come from.

When we got to where we had stopped to sit only a few minutes earlier, I noticed a bit of a bounce in his step. And a few minutes later, his pace increased.

"Well, that seems to be helping," I said, smiling at him.

"What?" he said, puzzled.

"The oxygen must be working. You're walking faster."

"Actually, I do feel like I can breathe a bit easier," he said, slightly surprised. We made our way to the other end of the thoroughfare and entered the warm building there. Here we continued browsing the indoor market while making our way back toward the truck. We met Jan and Wilma in the last building by the booth that sold windchimes. We laughed as we told them about our windchime adventure. Jan also commented that Jim was looking a bit better. Jim unzipped his jacket with a smile, "I have a little help. It works good."

Once outside the truck, I helped unhook Jim from the oxygen tank, and he climbed back into the driver's seat while I stowed away his oxygen tank under my seat behind him. Jim then took us to Listowel to show them where he used to work. Pulling into the parking lot, Jim called his friend Todd, one of the salesmen there. Todd came out for a visit as Jim and I rolled down the driver's side windows.

"Hey, buddy! How's it going!" asked Todd enthusiastically.

"Not bad for an old guy!" Jim said back, then quickly looked at me in the rear-view mirror. I said nothing, knowing he knew I recalled our earlier conversation about Joshua.

"What have you been up to?" Todd asked before introducing Jan and Wilma. After asking how things were at work, the topic went to pie, neither remembering who was buying who the next piece. From there, we drove toward home, showing off the cold Canadian winter landscape. After dinner, Jim took out the tile game Rummikub, asking if they had played it before.

"Oh yes, we have that game in Holland too. Let's play," Wilma said.

"Yes, she likes to win," Jan said in mock grumpiness. Thinking we wouldn't have to explain the rules, Jim dumped the game out of its box. Well, some rules were a little grey on both sides of the world, so we made up a few as we went. This was the go-to game throughout their visit. We played multiple games a day. Calvin and Josh would saunter over and sneak in a game or two from time to time. Occasionally we would change things up and play a game of golf on the Nintendo Wii, another of Jim's favourite games. But this was getting harder for him to play as swinging the "club" with both hands was painful. Josh tried to get him to play with just a flick of the wrist, but that wasn't real golf, in Jim's opinion. Other times, when I was cooking with Wilma, Jan would challenge Josh to a game of chess while Jim took a nap so he would be able to keep up with the activities. He didn't want to miss a thing.

Each morning and evening, Jan would stroll beside Jim as they made their way to the chicken condo to collect eggs and fill the feeders. Most days, Jim would sit on the feed sack while Jan would do the work, and they would talk like old friends.

The next day Jan and Wilma went to check out Stratford while Jim and I met with the nurse at home. The occupational therapist also came to talk to us about the Assistance Device Program. Jim could get a walker or wheelchair free for a month before we would have to rent one. She told us to look into the March of Dimes as she thought they helped if you had an income of $30,000 or less. She also encouraged us to look into the Ontario Renovates program for help with the bathroom renovations for Jim.

Jim drove the four of us to the Country Sisters restaurant outside of Listowel for lunch on Saturday. Jim stayed in the truck with Jan and Wilma while I went in to get us a table. As I stood in line, I texted them a running commentary. "Five people in front of me." "Oh, now there are two!" "The coconut cream pie looks good!"

When I finally secured a table, I met them at the door as Jim slowly progressed across the parking lot without his oxygen tank. It took all he had to get to the table. We stuffed him in the far corner of our booth to help keep his anxiety down. It felt odd to be the protector. He was always the one who boldly talked to people and was a visible presence in our family. Now he was shying away from people and felt insecure and vulnerable. It was another thing that was not my Jim, but it also helped me see that I could do this.

We enjoyed our delicious home-cooked Mennonite lunch of soup and fresh, flavourful sandwiches while we laughed, told stories, and lost all track of time. And a trip to Country Sisters would be incomplete without their signature pies which we slowly savoured.

As we finished, Jim leaned over to me and quietly asked, "Can you get a gift certificate for Todd when you pay the bill? We always took turns paying, and I'm pretty sure it was supposed to be my turn next. I don't think I will be able to do it again."

My heart sank as I scrambled to find other options, "What if I helped you, and we came back next week and met him here for lunch?"

"No, I'll just mail him a gift certificate, and he can take someone else," he said. We agreed on an amount, and I paid for lunch and purchased the gift certificate. I returned to find him laughing at something Jan had said. He eyed the certificate and mouthed a thank you as he worked his way back out of the booth. I walked slowly beside him and then helped him back into the truck's driver's seat. Once everyone was settled in, we went to visit our daughter Christina and her family in Mount Forest. We visited on one side of the room as they were on the other, trying to keep Wesley away from Papa and Grandma.

Sunday bloomed bright as we participated in church online again. But this time, it was nice to worship with others. After church, we headed to Nico's family in Exeter for another hard, socially-distanced visit. Again, I could see Jim struggling. He hated that we had to tell the kids they had to stay back. During this visit, Nico told Jim he had booked off work the week of March 14. He and Jodi had talked about it, and he would come to help Jim do some of the jobs Jim needed help with around the garage. Smiling, he asked Jim to start a list. Jim, thankful, started naming things he would put on the list.

Next, we headed to St. Marys to show off Nathan's family while having another socially-distanced visit. From there, Jim made a detour to Fawcett Tractor Supply, where he worked for more than fourteen years before starting at Premiere in 2014.

After a late lunch and a rest, Melissa took us on a tour of the Koskamp water buffalo farm where she worked. We laughed at the pig snorting buffalo, a new sight for our friends. On the way home, we toured Derek and Danielle's long laneway just down the road from us. Derek called, laughing; he asked what we were doing creeping around his place. We told him we were giving an outdoor tour since we couldn't come inside because his family was sick.

After a leisurely day at home, Jan and Wilma explored the lovely town of St. Marys while Jim and I headed off to London to talk with Dr. Logan, the chemo doctor. As we waited in the small waiting room, Jim was getting uncomfortable and asked me for one of the morphine pills I had in my purse for the pain. Downing it with the water in his ever-present water bottle, he laid his head back against the wall while stretching his long legs out toward the bed in the middle of the room. He closed his eyes. When she arrived and started talking, Jim jumped in the chair, having fallen asleep. After apologizing and waiting for him to get comfortable, she spent a good chunk of time with us.

"Would you like to see the latest scan of your chest, Mr. Schreuders? It might help to understand what is happening inside of you," she politely asked. As a home-schooling mom, I was eager to see and learn more about what was happening inside his body.

"No, I do not want to see it," he said hesitantly. I was shocked. I was not expecting that answer. Looking at him, I asked, "Why not?"

"I just don't think I want to see it," he said, knowing that this monster called cancer was moving aggressively through his body, conquering new territory, staking its claim. I reached for his hand. I realized that if he saw the scan he would have to admit how bad it was. That he wasn't getting better. I confessed to the doctor that I was interested. But it was up to him to decide.

"Can I show you the one with the fluid in it before we drained it?" she asked him, to which he agreed, probably more for my sake. She turned to the computer screen and keyboard mounted on the wall beside her and pulled up Jim's chart. Seeing this scan, he relaxed a little and allowed her to go to the more recent one. This one revealed that the mets were between the lung lining and were pushing the lung up. When you looked at the right lung, the healthier one, and compared it to the left one, it was easy to see that the left one didn't have room to expand. The tumours squished it up—way up—to half the size of his right lung. She explained that when the blood goes through the lung, it gathers oxygen to take with it throughout the rest of the body. This oxygenated blood helps keep all your organs alive and healthy. When your lung cannot expand, it cannot collect the needed oxygen. I pointed to the left bronchus tube, "It looks like the tumours are pushing this tube. Will it block the use of his lung?"

"Yes, it will. Actually, that is a good thing because then the blood won't flow through there; it will just go through the right lung to get more oxygen-enriched blood. Right now, the blood does not have a good supply of oxygen in it," she interpreted. This is what is causing his shortness of breath. It is also why he needs to use oxygen now when walking longer distances.

She then asked Jim about his thoughts and wishes regarding the end of life.

"I want to be home and not in a hospital. Is that what you mean?" he questioned.

"Do you want to be resuscitated if you stop breathing? We would like to know your wishes as they need to go into your paperwork."

"Well, right now, I still want them to try everything they can to keep me alive," he stated, a little frustrated.

"And they will, but Mr. Schreuders, this disease has exploded inside you. There is nothing more we can do except keep you comfortable. There is a medicine we can give you that will make you feel relaxed and comfortable." She turned to me, "But your family will see your body struggling. Mrs. Schreuders, I want you to know that he will not know that he is struggling." Tears ran down my cheeks as I tried to wipe them away. I fished in my pocket for a tissue. Dr. Logan reached over and handed me the small box of tissues next to her.

"Sorry," I mumbled, while drying my eyes, not wanting to visualize this future.

"There is nothing to be sorry about. This is a hard thing you are going through," she reassured me. She began to explain that there is only so much radiation a person can handle before it starts to do more damage than good. She then confirmed that the tumours were now immune to the radiation and that more were growing. We let that sink in. No more radiation; Jim was at his limit.

She explained three possible courses of chemo treatment. She told Jim that the first two would probably not be for him as they wouldn't give him the quality of life he wanted. He would probably have to be in the hospital and she knew that wasn't where he wanted to be. We were so thankful, sitting there, knowing that she was listening to what we were saying and taking it seriously. They were willing to work with us.

"Jim, you know that this isn't going away, right?" Jim understood. "We are just trying to keep you comfortable and maybe get you a bit more time. With this in mind, I would like to propose the third option, Gemcitabine." She chuckled, "We call it the old lady chemo because it is what we give old ladies. It's not as hard on the body. It has the possibility of making you tired or giving you an upset stomach, even nausea. But there is less chance of having these symptoms than with the other drug therapy options." She continued, "This is an intravenous drug that is given in a 28-day cycle. You would come in for treatment one day a week over the course of three weeks, followed by a week off. This can be continued for as long as it works. It should slow the growth of the tumours and possibly shrink some. You will have to keep an eye on your temperature at all times." Turning to me, she continued, "If it starts to go up a little, you can treat it with Tylenol. But, if it gets to 38 degrees or higher, don't take any Tylenol; just go straight to the emergency department. When we are finished here, the nurse will come in and give you a fever card with details about what drug he's taking and what to do. If you end up in the emergency department, you will need to give them this card. It will get you the right help faster."

Jim didn't want to give up trying, and this seemed like the best option. She agreed that if he did this, he and the rest of the family might feel like we didn't give up, and wouldn't regret later that we hadn't tried one more thing. Once we made this decision, she said Jim needed new antibiotics to cure the infection in his right lung that was causing his ongoing low-grade fever.

After our farewell, we waited for the nurse to come in with paperwork for Jim to sign, the fever card, and a script for the new antibiotics. The levofloxacin 750 mg was to be started that night, as he had finished the other antibiotics that morning.

Jim's phone rang as we climbed into the truck in the parking lot. It was Dr. Fortin's office. We were supposed to have had a phone meeting earlier with Dr. Fortin, but we missed it while talking with Dr. Logan. They were rescheduling it for two days from now.

On the way home, while formulating another email, we got a text from Jan, "I lost the car!" As we had to drive through St. Marys ourselves, I thought we should help him find it. Jim, on the other hand, said Jan and Wilma would be fine.

149

"Sure, you can say that because you are driving your truck. This is my car we are talking about," I joked. But seeing how tired he was, I didn't push it. I knew he just needed his chair.

After a nap, Pastor Martin came for another short visit. Jim talked about death and how we were coping with the reality of it all. Jim also told him how important it was that no one be turned away; he wanted anyone who wanted to visit to come visit. What that would look like, I didn't know. As I pondered this, Jan and Wilma had arrived home (with my car), and Pastor Martin left after praying with all of us.

Feeling rejuvenated after his nap and his chat with the minister, Jim wanted to visit Tavistock Premier to show Jan and Wilma where he worked. After introductions and the regular joking and teasing in the front office, Jim led the tour to the shop out back. He showed off some big tractors to Jan, both of them in their element, while Wilma and I stood back, having our own conversation. Then through the side door, behind Jim, came an old customer of his.

"Jim! I have not seen you around in a while. How are you?" the customer asked. I saw Jim hesitate.

"Well, to be honest, I'm not doing too well," Jim said honestly.

"Yeah, I heard you have cancer?"

"Yes, and it doesn't look too good. So, how's the family?" Jim changed the subject with a skill I knew he didn't realize he had. I was proud of him.

We were sad as we got up the next morning, knowing it was the last day we had with Jan and Wilma. To cheer everyone up, Joshua and I pulled out a small Dairy Queen ice cream birthday cake for Jan, as we would miss his special day tomorrow. Jim gave him a gift, a John Deere sweatshirt he, not so secretly, bought yesterday. Going into the hall, he also took one of his many new ball caps and gave it to Jan. Pulling on the shirt and securing the hat on his head, Jan said he wanted a photo of the two of them since Jim was already wearing his John Deere sweatshirt and hat. Later we laughed at the picture. They could have passed for brothers. Deep down, of course, they were.

After playing another round of chess with Joshua, the boys said their goodbyes, and we headed toward Niagara. We stopped to see my godparents, Keith and Ann, to say hi before they headed to Florida for a vacation. I offered to help Jim with the oxygen tank, but he said he should be fine. Feeling that the door was not too far away, he figured he could get there if he went slowly. He had already instructed that we were not to stay long, just say hi. Once they saw us, they ushered us in the door, where we finished re-introductions from thirty-two years earlier. All the while, Jim moved slower the closer he got to the door. He was grateful to just slide into the welcoming bench that sat just inside the door. With great hesitation, he returned Ann's hug and Keith's pat on the shoulder. Even though he was happy to see them, as they were to see him, he still worried about catching something. After the short visit and once Jim regained some strength, we headed out and made our way to Desiree's family's house.

Desiree introduced her family as we stayed distanced again. Both Desiree and I could see that Jim wanted a better visit but struggled with how to do that. All I knew to do was follow his lead. When he asked Desiree to give them a bit of a tour, that's what we did.

After the all-too-short visit, we headed to my parents' place, where Jan and Wilma would stay for three more days. During the remaining days, they would be doing touristy things with my younger brother James whom they had gotten to know when they were here for our wedding. My mom invited my brother's and sister's families for a pizza dinner. Sitting distanced from each other, we enjoyed our visit while joking and laughing together.

Our daughter Elly was staying here with her grandparents while she was in school. I saw her watching her dad from across the room. How I wanted to comfort her, hug her. But I knew she was not in our "circle." Later she told me she was waiting to follow Jim's lead like I was. So going out to the garage and unpacking Jan and Wilma's suitcases before we left, she followed, hovering in the background.

With the luggage unloaded, we loaded my grandma's wheelchair and the shower chair into the back of the truck. We gave long, tearful goodbyes to Jan and Wilma, holding on for as long as possible and then a few more minutes. It was so hard saying goodbye under these circumstances. Harder than I ever thought was possible, each of us in a puddle of our own tears. Then Jim noticed Elly and went over to her. He hugged her, breaking her resolve, as she cried in her daddy's arms. Finally pulling back, he looked down at her and gave a weak smile with his red-rimmed eyes.

He turned and walked to the truck, "Come on, Mama. Time to go." He attempted to be cheerful. I was sad as I got in beside him. We began our two-hour-long drive home in a melancholy atmosphere.

"That was hard. Harder than I thought it would be," he divulged, breaking the thick silence in the truck a while later. I quietly agreed, and we began to talk about the visit. How good it had been to reminisce about the past thirty-two years. Coming up with "remember when" stories to share and just laugh. Laughing was so, so good! It relieved the tension that had built up between us, and our kids. Laughing was something we needed to do more of.

Think about it

Have you looked back at your life lately? Have you taken some time
to look back and marvel at God's faithfulness in your life? Maybe
there were times when you didn't have money to pay for a need,
but it worked out. Or perhaps you had distress or brokenness in
your life that God brought you through. Now look ahead and trust
Him, for He cares for you. "*Humble yourselves, therefore, under
God's mighty hand, that he may lift you up in due time. Cast all your
anxiety on him because he cares for you*" (1 Peter 5:6–7).

Friendships Are Important

THE NEXT MORNING, things were back to our new normal. After we checked on the chickens together, Jim received a text from Jan, "Hello Brother. How are you today?" This continued over the coming days. Every morning Jan would text "Hello Brother," and it would be followed by a short conversation on the weather, chickens, or some other everyday event. Friendships, not only Jan and Wilma's but so many others during these past months, were so dear to Jim, to us. Jim would put all caution aside and hug his dear friends. So many of those hugs came with tears, but he was so past being a "tough guy." He wanted to be the "real guy." He wanted to be the guy who let those around him know how much he cared for them.

At 10:30 am, Dr. Fortin called Jim to discuss any hesitations or questions he might have. First, he asked her if surgery was possible, as he understood radiation was no longer an option. Next, she explained that she had looked at his CT scans from February 2 to February 20 and noticed that the disease was progressing quite a bit. On this scan, she could still see some fluid on the base of the left lung, but the thickening all along the wall was more concerning. Jim pointed out that he felt pressure in this area and was wondering if she could just cut out the lung, as people have been known to live with one lung. Finally, she graciously explained to us, in terms we could understand, what was happening inside Jim.

"Think of your lungs as a bed sponge, the foam layer you put on top of your bed. The tumours are like cement. The cement coats the sponge, taking over. Regarding your question Mr. Schreuders, yes, we can take out the lung and tumours. I know how and I can. But we, as doctors, have learned from the past that this procedure is very manipulating and does not give patients the quality of life they would like. The patients who have had this surgery do not live as long, and are in much more pain than those who do not have the surgery."

Hearing this information, Jim realized this was definitely not on his list of things to do. He thanked her, letting her know he was very grateful for her time and all the work she had done for him. She appreciated his kind words and wished Jim all the best in the days ahead.

Jim found he needed to call people and initiate conversations as people didn't want to bother him. People were always glad to talk to him but didn't always know what to say. During those long days he just wanted to speak to someone in order to break up his every day. And so did I. It helped us be open and not to slip back into tiptoeing around each other.

Our neighbour and friend, Nick, came over to visit often, and Jim roped him into playing multiple games of Rummikub. I was thankful for someone else to take my spot as his opponent. I needed time to do some meal prep, baking, and other house-work, especially with Jim inviting more people to come visit. People were starting to come and go every day, one in the morning and another in the afternoon. So many that I can't remember them all. But it sure helped to pass the time, whether playing board games, card games, or simply visiting.

"It's coming soon," he would say more often now, followed by a new thing he had lost that day. Whether it was going out to see his chickens, which he now had our youngest Josh do for him, or the ability to play Wii golf with the boys, as this caused too much pain on his left side, he had lost so much. It was disheartening for me to watch, yet we could mourn these losses together. He was trying to find the good in each loss. What good can come from this? Well, we had time alone together when Josh was out with the chickens or a laugh when Jim talked to him in the chicken condo through his phone. And the good in not playing Wii? He didn't have to lose anymore, even though he rarely did lose. As he gave us this play-by-play, he also prepared us for the future.

On Friday night he told me he wanted to take the two youngest boys out for lunch the next day. He knew we had spent so much time with Jan and Wilma, leaving those two boys behind. He wanted to spend time with them and decided to take them to his favourite lunchtime restaurant, Country Sisters.

"You know that's not where they want to go," I said, already envisioning the teen-age drama that would ensue. "They serve soup and sandwiches, which they think is boring."

"Well, I don't want to go out to KFC or something like that. They can do that any day. I want to take them out somewhere different, somewhere special. Think about it and let me know if you come up with something else." That night, I thought about it, concluding that they don't always need to get what they want; they have to explore different things. Country Sisters would be where they went with their dad. So in the morning we told the boys we were taking them out.

On the way to Country Sisters, we all sang along with Jim. We sang songs from the late 70s and early 80s, even the high and low parts. Again, Jim waited in the truck while I stood in line. Getting a booth in the back this time, we enjoyed a delicious meal of soup, sandwiches… and pie, of course. Jim told the boys, just like in the good old days, he wanted to take them to Listowel Premier. He wanted to show them the new renovations that were done since he used to take them to work with him.

One of the parts guys offered to take us on a tour. I offered to get Jim his oxygen, but he was determined to do this without it. After Jim placed a card with the Country Sister's gift certificate on Todd's desk, we toured the new building, moving slowly. Then we walked across the parking lot to the old building, which had been renovated into a showroom. The boys found it fascinating trying to figure out where Dad's office used to be as the shiny new floor and new walls gave away no hints. As we returned to the new building, I noticed Jim was waning. I was worried as I saw him pushing himself to do this for the boys. He made it back to the truck on his own power and was happy to have given the boys a day to remember.

A day of worship. How we wished we could be in person with all our church family. This day Jim and I sat side by side because standing with the congregation was too much for him. We again felt the songs we had sung for years in the church with a new deep, personal meaning. They are not just words on a page or screen anymore. They are not just beautiful melodies. Today as those in the church sang "Yet Not I But Through Christ In Me,"[10] we at home were sobbing. These words were what we had been clinging to each and every day. We needed this reminder that we can't do it on our own, but through Christ in us, we can.

After church, noticing that it was getting warmer outside, Jim wanted to get some fresh air and sit on his motorcycle. After the emotional service, I just felt I needed to be close to him.

"Can I come out with you, or did you need time alone?" I asked.

"You can come," he said. With a smile he added," We can talk about our *relationship*," dragging out the last word. We both laughed, as this is something I always wanted to do. Sweeping up my hand, he pulled me with him out to the garage. I helped him open the heavy overhead garage door so we could let the sun and fresh air in. He went over to his motorcycle, pulling his sleeve down over his wrist; he used it to dust off the dashboard and seat. Then, with his left hand on the handlebar, he swung his right leg over the bike. He started playing with the radio, checking to make

---

[10] Jonny Robinson, Michael Farren, and Rich Thompson, "Yet Not I But in Christ Through Me," CityAlight Music, 2018.

sure his favourite cassette tape, *Promise Keepers: The Making of a Godly Man*, was in. He turned the key and started the music, singing his heart out with the song, "We Shall Overcome/We Have Overcome."[11] Taking out my phone from where I was sitting on the lawnmower on the other side of the garage, I took a short video of him as my vision blurred. I needed this memory to stay forever. I needed to remember my godly husband, the father of my ten children. Later that day, I posted it on the FamJam chat as I knew some of my children would treasure this memory too.

When he was done singing his song, we talked about the weather. It was so much warmer than when Jan and Wilma were here. Hatching a plan, he had me help push the motorcycle outside, where the snow was melting on the driveway. In only a sweatshirt, he pulled on his helmet and pretended to be riding his bike while I took a photo. Laughing, he sent it to Jan, telling him the weather was so beautiful that he went out for a ride. Little did we know this would be the last time he would sit on his beloved bike.

That afternoon we made our way to see his parents. We knew that it was not possible for Dad to come to visit him, so he wanted to make sure he went there as much as he could. He wanted to show his dad and mom that he was okay. Maybe if they saw him every week, then it would be a gradual thing, and they wouldn't notice. Yes, he was chipper, and he still had his sense of humour, which we were all thankful for, but I knew they saw what I saw. I could see it in his mother's sad eyes. The way his dad looked at him, waiting for him to tell him it was not so.

That night Jim tried keeping his oxygen on to see if it made any difference. It seemed to help, so he decided to continue keeping his oxygen on at night. But he still preferred not to during the day.

---

[11] "We Shall Overcome/We Have Overcome," track 11 on Maranatha! Promise Band, *Promise Keepers – The Making of a Godly Man,* Maranatha Music, 1997.

Tying up Loose Ends

JIM CALLED THE lawyer and asked if there was anything we should do to get our affairs in order. He wanted to make things as easy as possible for me when he was gone. The lawyer thought the only thing that would be helpful would be to move all the vehicles into my name. So today, we would make that our main task, right after picking up the long-term disability papers from Dr. Thornton's office. This five-page form was now an additional twenty-five pages when we picked it up. It contained all Jim's medical records from all his doctor's visits related to his cancer. Jim was excited about his new reading project.

Afterward, at the St Marys license office, we were told to go to the town office and get a form signed and witnessed, stating that Jim was gifting me his truck. Since the car was already in my name, we didn't need to worry about that one. We drove to the office just south of town. After strapping on Jim's oxygen tank, we made our way into the building. After everything was signed and witnessed, we made our way back to the license office, west of town. Jim didn't want to get out and be bothered with the oxygen tank, so he asked if I would just run in and do the paperwork. If he needed to sign anything I could bring it out to the truck. So I went in alone. We began filling out the paperwork. When I realized he didn't sign one of the papers, I ran out to him, then back in. I was thankful there was no one else there at the time, as I needed to run out a second time for another autograph before we were finished.

Returning to the truck, I climbed in, not really sure if I should say anything. This was *his* truck. He loved this truck. This was just one more thing he was losing. As I closed the passenger door behind me, Jim turned in his seat to face me.

"Mrs. Schreuders?" he said seriously.

"Yes?" not sure whether to take him seriously or not.

"May I please drive *your* truck?" he said as the corners of his mouth went up.

"I guess. As long as you are careful," I replied, letting out the breath I didn't realize I was holding in as we both burst out laughing.

Think about it

Do you have something that you treasure here on Earth? Something that, if lost or destroyed, would be devastating to you? The treasures of heaven far outweigh any earthly item. *"Set your mind on things above, not on earthly things"* (1 Peter 5:6–7).

"I feel like I'm going downhill fast," Jim told Dr. Thornton over the phone. "I have pain in my left side. My back hurts today, which I haven't had before. And I have shortness of breath even when I am sitting."

"Are you using your oxygen?"

"Yes, almost all day and night."

"How is your mood, Jim?" a question she would often ask him now.

"For the most part, I'm good. But at night, when I'm lying in bed, I get anxious about not being able to breathe. It was very bad the other day when I came back from feeding the chickens. That was a horrible feeling. I don't want that again."

Wanting to let her know how serious this was for him, I added, "It has always been a fear of his, even before any of this started. He has always been afraid of feeling like he can't breathe."

"Well, Jim, when a person's oxygen gets below 80 percent, it can feel like they are drowning. But we have medication to help you not feel that way. This is why we need to keep track of your oxygen levels. The morphine should also help," she explained. He said it did help, having taken more at the four-hour intervals to help him breathe better. "Do you ever take your oxygen levels when you are short of breath, Jim?"

"No, we just do them in the morning and at night. Should we be?" he asked.

"It might not be a bad idea. Then we have a record of it. Can you tell me what they were when you did record it, Joanne?"

"This morning, it was 88 percent. Yesterday, March 7, it was 91 percent in the morning and 92 percent in the evening. On March 6 it was 94 percent in the morning and 90 percent in the evening. March 5 was 97 percent in the morning and 92 percent in the evening." She had us take his oxygen readings while we were talking. They were 92 percent with two litres of oxygen. She had Jim take off the oxygen for a bit and then redo the reading. It was 84 percent.

We went on to discuss the shakes and shivers he would get every night before bed. We didn't know why, but we could count on them coming. I would help him get dressed and get him settled in bed, and he would shake and shiver. His teeth chattered. So I would climb in beside him. Wrapping my leg around his, I would snuggle close and rub his arms, trying to warm him with my body heat. I also noticed that his hands and feet would sometimes twitch throughout the day. We didn't know if this meant something, but we thought we should tell her.

With all the morphine in his system, it was only a given that his bowels were having a hard time, even with the meds for that exact purpose.

"How is your appetite?" she asked.

"I'm not very hungry," he said.

"That can also be because you have decreased the Dex. When was your last one?"

"Last Thursday," I said, looking back in the brown notebook.

"Is he still confused?" she asked me.

"No, that seems to have improved too," I said, somewhat relieved.

"I think I need to go back on the Dex," he petitioned. Inside I sighed. It had been a struggle to get him off, to clear his head. With all those drugs I was still carrying in my purse, he was now only on the morphine.

"Jim, if you feel that is what you need to do, then I will write you a script and send it off," she said.

"Yes, please," he requested, while his shoulders sagged. I knew he felt more energetic when he was on the Dex. He wanted that energy back, and I couldn't take that from him.

"Can you tell me about your meeting with Dr. Logan? I don't have any notes here from her yet," she said. We told her about the chemo Jim was hopefully going on soon. While we talked about this, Jim would start the conversation, but then he would get winded, motioning me to finish.

"I want to start this, as soon as possible (pause for breath) because I feel like (breath) it will be too late (breath) if I wait longer," Jim informed her with not much emotion.

"I will call Dr. Logan tomorrow and find out what the plan is for chemo if you would like," she asked.

"That would be great," Jim said, perking up a bit.

"I will also have to discuss with her if you can actually be on Dex if you are on the chemo drug," she informed Jim.

She then informed us that her family got good news and was going to celebrate with a trip to Hawaii during March Break. We were excited for her and the time she would be able to spend with her family. We were sure her job didn't allow for much treasured family time. She told us she was working on getting another doctor, Dr. Thomas, who would be looking after us for the week she was gone.

After a conversation about how our kids were handling Jim's situation, she said goodbye with a promise to contact Dr. Logan in the morning. She also requested that the nurse call her when she came to visit the next morning.

After the appointment we visited with our friends Stan and Joanne in the dining room. Unlike our last visit with them, Jim was not able to tell all the stories he wanted to. He would start, then look at me and say, "You tell them." Sometimes he had me go get a photo album to show pictures. He was happy, and content for the most part. But then that line would come again.

"I'm so glad I have Joanne here with me (breath) helping me go through this. (breath) I couldn't do it without her. (breath) I just feel bad that I can't (breath) be here for her someday." So many breathing breaks.

"Jim, do you really think you have taken care of your family all these years?" asked Stan, looking straight at Jim. Jim looked at him, trying to understand his question. "Jim, you have never been in control of what your family does or doesn't do. You can't keep them all safe. God does that!" He waited while that sunk in. "Jim, when you are gone, He will still care for your family. Just like He has been doing all these years." He said this matter-of-factly.

Jim looked at Stan, realizing that he had been looking at this all wrong. A smile broke out on his face, "You're right. He has, hasn't He!" Even after they left a bit later, Jim still sat there thinking about Stan's wise words. Those words, I could see, made a physical impact on him. He appeared to be happier, as he realized we would be okay. God had us.

The next morning, we decided to sit down and work together on that year's income tax report. In the past, I have always kept the books, but Jim did the income tax. He wanted to teach me how to do it. So, sitting down together, side by side, we began the online tax form.

Jim's phone rang, interrupting our data entry. It was a Dr. Thomas. He introduced himself and said that he had just talked with Dr. Thornton and would be taking over for her while she was on holiday. It was only a short call, just for introductions. Once we hung up, we moved back to the income tax form, only to be interrupted by another call on Jim's phone.

Jim answered the phone rather brightly, while still sitting beside me at the dining room table. Dr. Logan's voice came through the speaker.

"Good morning, Jim! I just got off the phone with Dr. Thornton. She says you are having trouble breathing?" Jim confirmed that he was. "I wish I could have this conversation with you in my office, face to face, but this is probably easier for you," she said sympathetically.

"Yes, this is fine," Jim reassured her.

"Well, can you tell me what is going on with you?"

"It is harder to breathe. (breath) I can barely make it (breath) from my bed to the bathroom. (breath) Or from the bathroom to my chair. (breath) My left side is uncomfortable. (breath) I just don't think I have much time," he informed her.

She went on to explain how the rapidly growing disease was resistant to radiation. Because of this, she was pretty sure it wouldn't react to the chemo. She believed the side effects of this chemo would affect his quality of life, particularly by making him more tired.

"I would strongly advise that you do not do the chemo treatment, Mr. Schreuders. I do not think it will help you in any way, but actually make things worse," she put forward.

"Can I think about this?" he asked.

"Absolutely. You, or your wife, or even Dr. Thornton, can call me back with your decision."

"I just want to thank you for being honest with us about the chemo. It means a lot to us that you are not pushing it on us, but just informing us of all the options," he said, genuinely thankful.

"Mr. Schreuders, may I just say how refreshing it is to hear how well you are taking this news?"

"Well, I have lived fifty-four great years. God has blessed me beyond belief. I have no regrets, and I am truly thankful," he said honestly.

"Mr. Schreuders, it amazes me that you can say that. You are handling this so well. Keep it up," she encouraged before saying her farewells and letting us know that she was still available if we needed someone to talk to about any of the treatments. As Jim turned off the phone, I backed up my chair a little, attempting to face him better. I reached over while encouraging him to turn and face me.

Taking his face between my two hands, I said with tears spilling over, "And *that* is doing it well, Jim."

Taking a minute and looking into my eyes, he asked, "Do you really think so?" He was not quite sure of himself.

"I *know* so," I said, kissing him. He pulled me into an embrace. After a moment, we both sat back, swiping at our tears. I turned, once again, to face the computer screen. Jim got up and went to sit on his chair behind me, promising to answer any questions I had.

Think about it

Do you feel like you are insignificant and can't be used by God? Do you feel like you have limitations or inabilities? Do you think you are imperfect or flawed? Then you are just what the Lord needs. God sees opportunity where we see weakness and obstacles. *"But he said to me, 'My grace is sufficient for you, for my power is made perfect in weakness.' Therefore I will boast all the more gladly about my weaknesses, so that Christ's power may rest on me. That is why, for Christ's sake, I delight in weaknesses, in insults, in hardships, in persecutions, in difficulties. For when I am weak, then I am strong"* (2 Corinthians 12:9–10).

After lunch, his nurse Andrea arrived to do his vitals. We talked casually about things happening in our families while enjoying her company. Andrea called Dr. Thornton, remembering she wanted to talk to us.

"So, I talked to Dr. Thomas this morning," Dr. Thornton stated.

"He called here this morning," we chuckled.

"Okay, that was quick. I also talked with Dr. Logan."

"Yes, she called here too," Jim laughed.

"Well then, what did you guys decide about the chemo?" she asked. Jim explained that she was giving us time to think about it, but he was pretty sure he didn't want to do it. Dr. Thornton agreed to contact Dr. Logan and let her know his decision.

"I have a few questions. (breath) First, can I start the Dex up again?" Jim asked.

"Since you have decided not to do the chemo, we won't need to worry about them working against each other. So yes, we can start it. You had a second question?"

"Yes. Can I have more coffee?"

"Oh, yes, definitely! Have whatever you want," she chuckled.

"More pie?" he said with raised eyebrows. We were all laughing now.

"Yes, Jim, more pie!" she said.

"Mama, did you hear that? (breath) More pie!"

"Yes, dear, I heard. I'll get right on it," I said, rolling my eyes in mock exasperation.

Dr. Thornton then went on to discuss planning and prioritizing visitors, which I don't think she realized we were doing already. Jim smiled at me, as I realized he was thinking the same thing.

"Jim is anxious about people bringing COVID into the house," I verbalized. She then reviewed the COVID prevention measures we could have in place here at home. We went over things like washing hands, sanitizing, keeping distance, and wearing masks. We were to ensure people did not visit if they didn't feel well.

Again, Jim said he felt he didn't have much time. She said that she had to agree with him, that he wouldn't have as much time as they had hoped. We discussed additional meds that could keep him comfortable in the coming days. One was Ritalin, to help give him more energy. But for now, she felt the Dex would do that.

"When your oxygen is low, Jim, you can turn up the tank. It will help you, too," she informed us.

"The lady that set up the oxygen stressed we were to keep it at two litres." I was a little perplexed.

"It's okay to put it all the way up if you have to. The goal is to keep his oxygen above 90. And right now the levels are between 85 and 90." I agreed as Andrea gave us an encouraging nod. Dr. Thornton then took a few minutes to talk to Jim about the DNR form (Do not resuscitate).

"Jim, we have talked about this form before. Have you decided yet what you want to do?" she asked.

Sighing, he said, "Yes, I will sign it."

"If it's any consolation, Jim, I think you are making the right choice," Dr. Thornton said caringly, with Andrea nodding her agreement. Dr. Thornton then talked with Andrea about some medical stuff before she came back with the form for Jim to sign.

"I feel like I'm signing my life away," Jim said.

"Jim, I'm sure it feels like that, but it is a good thing you are doing. This way your family is not forced to make the decision. You are giving them peace of mind," Andrea encouraged. They were right. It did give me peace of mind. I didn't have to make that call, with the thought that I might be going against his wishes. I was very thankful that he made that hard call for me.

"I know, but it still feels like it," he said sadly. I reached over and held him.

Later, as I showed Andrea to the door, Kate from occupational therapy arrived for her appointment. Kate had also brought some cushions for Jim to try on his chair. He picked one that was comfortable and worked for him. She then had Jim sit in the wheelchair from my parents and adjusted it for him.

"Are the newer wheelchairs lighter," he asked.

"Yes, they would be easier to maneuver and put in and out of the car," she informed him.

"Maybe we should rent a newer one," he said, looking at me. "It'll be easier for you to push me around." I was not so sure I wanted to rent one if we had this one. Would we go out enough to justify a lighter one? This one was fine for in the house. "It would be handy if we go on the St. Marys trail, (breathe) it's wheelchair assessable." While he said this he smiled that smile that made me want to give him the world. I gave in. Kate did up the paperwork. She also ordered a commode and an air mattress for the bed to help prevent bedsores since he was spending more time sitting and sleeping than walking and standing.

At one point, Jim again stressed that he didn't want me to turn anyone away.

"If they want to come to visit, let them," he demanded.

"What if it is too much?" I asked him.

"Nope, let them come."

"Let's come up with a sign that you can give me when it's too much."

"No!"

"Jim, please," I begged, "If it becomes too much, then I can gently encourage our guests to leave."

"Okay, I will agree to a sign, but I don't want anyone to be turned away," he stressed.

In between visits, if he was not napping, he played Rummikub. By this time, the kids were sick of the game, but he could keep playing. He roped me into playing whenever he could. I remember thinking at one point while waiting for him to take his turn that it was like we were waiting for death to come. Life seemed so meaningless at this point. I was thankful when people came to help pass the time. I will admit it, Jim was right; we needed people. The reminiscing was so good for our souls, laughing at all the good memories.

Coming Home

ON THURSDAY WE started the day by doing Jim's vitals in his chair. I laid down the blood pressure cuff and oxygen sensor on the dining room table as we reviewed the income tax return, double-checking my work before submitting it online. During this checking, Jim discovered he could apply for a disability tax credit. He started to fill out the lengthy paperwork online. Figuring this would take a while, I told him I would take a quick shower while he worked on the form. Nodding his agreement, I headed for the shower.

Joshua came running to the door, as I finished showering and dressing around 10:00 am.

"Dad needs you!" I ran to the dining room and found him sitting on a chair, leaning on the table, with the oxygen sensor on his finger, a weak, helpless look on his face. I looked down to read the oxygen levels, 70 percent. Trying to hold back my panic, I soothingly talked to him as I called the nurses. He reached out for my hand and held tight. No answer.

Wanting to help him breathe, I rubbed his back and held his hand while quietly saying, "It's okay, just breathe. You got this. In. Out. In. Out." Why were the nurses not calling? Lord, help us! Bring his oxygen back up. I don't know what else to do, Lord.

"You're doing good, dear. I love you. Just breathe." Maybe I was saying it for me too? My phone dinged with a message at 10:10 am. I looked down to see it was Dr. Thornton, "Thinking of you today. Please try to get some couple time too—sometimes it is hard to be both caregiver and nurse and simply spouse. You are such a strong, inspiring woman. Wish your path wasn't this one."

Not even registering the message, my fingers flew a message back to her, "You are an answer to prayer. Jim's oxygen just dipped to 70. It's up again to the low 80s. Is there anything I can do for him?"

"Turn up the O2 on the concentrator to five. Let me know what his O2 rises to," came the quick reply. "SubQ morphine will help with air hunger which he will have at 80 percent or lower—it is a terrifying feeling. Please ask the nurse to call me or send me the nurse's number. He needs a SubQ port put in, and there should be an injectable narcotic in SRK... Injectable will take away air hunger faster. I'll call you in a sec. If the nurse can't reach me on my cell, have her call me..."

"He is at 93 percent but feeling lightheaded."

"Can you check his blood pressure and please send me the nurse's number as soon as you can." I sent her the number and the extension.

"119/72. Pulse 95," I was happy to see his pulse was going down.

"107/67. Pulse 91," I messaged a few minutes later.

"Great. Your presence with him may be the 'treatment he needs' while feeling lightheaded. I think it should pass now that the O2 is up." We continued to message about getting another oxygen machine that would go up to ten pounds instead of the one we had that only went up to five pounds.

As Jim improved and got enough oxygen, he could talk again. He told me that he had been feeling well. He went to put a book on the shelf after he hit print for the disability form. He noticed the printer was out of paper and sat on the chair to get paper from the bottom shelf to refill the printer. This action took his breath away. When he got up to go to his recliner to rest, he could only reach the other side of the table in front of the laptop.

Jim again said it wouldn't be much longer. He said we should call Desiree and tell her she needs to come home now and not wait until her scheduled visit next Thursday.

"But my kids all have colds. I don't want to make it worse for you, Dad." We could hear the tears in her voice over the phone line.

"It doesn't matter anymore, Sweet Pea (his special nickname for her). Just come. Wear masks if it makes you feel better. Just come." We cried with Desiree as she promised to figure out something and to come as soon as possible.

Jim agreed to let me get him into the old wheelchair to make the move across the room to his recliner. From then on, he used the wheelchair to get from point A to point B, as any movement seemed to take his oxygen levels down. When his friend and neighbour Nick messaged, asking if he could visit, Jim encouraged him to come. He also apologized for not having the energy to play a game. Nick assured him he was fine with just sitting and visiting.

The doorbell rang that afternoon and a gentleman from Ontario Home Health was there with another oxygen machine that would reach ten pounds. It also came with another plastic bag of different masks. One was the regular clear one that would cover his nose and mouth. But the one they would like him to try was light green and had a small bag attached to the bottom. This one would continuously have good oxygenated air for him to breathe. We were told it was the best of all the masks.

Later that afternoon, Christina came for a visit with her two kids. Shock and worry registered on her face. Papa smiled as he reached for the baby and pulled her to his chest while reclining comfortably in his chair. Snuggling with his youngest grandbaby, he kept busy fussing over her. Sitting close to her dad, Christina told him she was supposed to do a Scentsy show out by Toronto. She asked him if she should cancel and just stay home, closer to him. He said he was good for now and that she should do her show. She promised she would return Sunday after the show was finished.

While they were here occupying Jim, I got a message from Dr. Thornton about the new oxygen machine and masks she ordered for Jim. She wanted to ensure we were well taken care of as she would be gone with her family on vacation. "And wanted to say sorry I won't be around for ten days. To me, it feels like I'm abandoning your family in a time of need. I'm sorry I can't be there."

I messaged back, "Do not feel bad. Just enjoy every minute with your husband and kids. Give them lots of hugs and hold them tight."

That evening Nico and Jodi visited with the kids after we had finished dinner. While I cleaned up, Jim sat in the wheelchair at the table, talking with Nico. He started fidgeting with the length of the oxygen tube. Soon he had it in two loops that looked like glasses. Holding them up to his face, he started making faces at the grandkids, causing them to giggle.

"Oh, Papa, you are so funny," said little Allie.

Our friends Jane and Herb arrived a little after 8:30 pm. Jane sometimes sings with a praise team in our church and Jim was so looking forward to having them over and singing together. I suggested maybe putting it off as he had a rough morning, but he would have none of it.

Using the song playlist Jane had made for Jim on her phone and the song sheets she had printed, we started singing while Nico's Allie and Graham danced with Christina's Wesley. Our son Nathan came in and sat watching Dad enjoying himself immensely. We sang song after song for almost an hour until we could see Jim's eyelids getting heavy.

Little did we know that Christina had told her siblings that Dad really was not doing well. Some thought she was exaggerating as the last they talked to him, he was fine, "Not bad for an old guy." Desiree told of her call with us that morning. After Elly had driven from Niagara to Guelph, going to Bible study with Melissa, they headed to our house to see for themselves. As they entered the house, they heard us singing, "Amazing Grace." Not knowing what to expect, they were anxious walking into the room. Upon slowly entering, they saw a thinner, weaker Dad sitting in a wheelchair. With an oxygen tube under his nose, smiling from ear to ear with tears glistening in his eyes, he tried to sing, but the lack of oxygen made it difficult. When he saw the girls, his hand flew in the air, "Hey! My girls are here!" his smile grew bigger.

When the singing was done, and Herb and Jane were getting ready to leave, our daughter-in-law, Jodi, asked if I could talk to her for a minute in the hall. She waved to Nico to join us. Once in the hall, she said, "Nico and I have a question we need to ask you. We are expecting, and we don't know if we should tell Dad." Oh, I was not expecting to hear that news. I was so excited! So excited I didn't hear the second part of Jodi's question. "We just don't know if it would make him too sad to know he won't meet this little one."

"Oh, you just *have* to tell him. He will be so excited! He needs this good news!" I said as I gave Jodi and Nico a big hug. When we returned to the dining room where Jim sat, Jodi let Allie and Graham know that it was time to go and say goodbye. I watched as Jodi hugged Jim and, with a smile, said, "And just so you know, you are hugging two." Jim sat up straighter, grabbed Jodi's hand, looking into her eyes, making sure he heard her right.

Then he looked at Nico, "You're having a baby?" Nico and Jodi nodded with big smiles on their faces. Jodi straightened and rubbed her belly, "Yep!"

Jim pumped his hand into the air, and with a whoop, he said, "That makes a dirty dozen!"

That night as we lay in bed, I could hear the smile in Jim's voice as he talked about this new little beautiful person that God was sending to Nico and Jodi. He knew he would never see this little one, but he was still so excited for them. Together we prayed for this little one and all our other grandchildren. We prayed that the Lord would bless them and keep them in His care. We prayed that someday they would also know the Lord and make Him their personal saviour.

Friday, we got up, thanking God for another day together. After breakfast, Jim and I did devotions. Jim answered Jan's "Good morning, brother!" text. I then helped him get cleaned up and dressed for the day. Afterward I went out to do his chicken chores. Later that morning, our friends Anton and Karen came for a visit and to play games. Again, the game of choice for Jim was Rummikub. After playing a few rounds, we decided to visit a bit. Jim had been telling them about the long-term disability form, and asked me to fetch it. He wanted to show them something in the twenty-five pages Dr. Thornton added to the form with all his medical records. As he leafed through the pages, the rest of us continued our conversation.

Suddenly, the arm that propped Jim's head up slipped off the table, causing his upper body to bounce like a ball. Startled, he looked up at us.

"Are you okay?" we asked.

"Oh, yeah!" he said, not missing a beat. "I was just reading this piece here," he said, locating his place on the paper before him. "I was pleased to speak to Mr. Schreuders on the phone today. This pleasant fifty-four-year-old gentleman ..." Looking back up at us, he continued, "She called me a pleasant gentleman. Never been called that before. Guess my head got a little big and heavy after reading that. I couldn't keep it up." He smiled. We couldn't help but laugh, and he laughed right along with us.

Jim napped after they left, before Desiree and her family arrived. When they arrived, Andrew, Eva, and Peter gave Papa hugs and were excited to try out Papa's wheelchair. Piling on, they had their dad, Joey, push them around while Papa watched, smiling from his chair. After a couple of hours, Joey and the kids said goodbye to Papa and Desiree before heading home. Joey and his family agreed to help with the kids again, so Desiree could stay as long as she needed.

After dinner, Desiree and Elly were playing a game of Rummikub with Jim. Well into the game, Jim was waiting for the girls to take their turns. He sat in his wheelchair at the end of the dining room table with his head propped in his hand. The girls looked up to see Jim slowly picking up tiles from the pickup pile and turning them over in front of him.

"What are you doing, Dad?" the girls asked as he began falling asleep in his wheelchair.

"Mom, I think Dad needs to go for a nap. He is not playing right." Once they rolled his wheelchair over, I transferred him into his recliner.

"I keep burping. Can you get me some of that Gas-X?" he asked me. I went to the medicine cupboard in the kitchen and came back with the pill. He looked up at me and questioned, "Is this safe to take?"

"Yes. You have had it before," I said, a bit baffled at his question.

"Can I see the box? I want to make sure." I came back with the box and handed it to him. He turned the box over in his hands and adjusted the position to find the right spot to read it through his multifocal glasses. A minute later he said, "Yep, it's good," and handed me the box as giggles irrupted from the girls.

Andrea arrived around 8:00 that night. She strongly suggested Jim have a catheter put in.

"No. Those things are so uncomfortable. I can get to the bathroom with Joanne's help." So, every time I moved him we had to crank up the oxygen tank as his oxygen levels would drop.

Andrea then put a port in his stomach, which Dr. Thornton had ordered, to attach the morphine pump that had arrived earlier that day. Whenever he felt short of breath, he could push the button (the bolus button) and it would release the morphine. It was attached to a mini computer which kept track of how many times he pushed the button, even though it only released the set amount. With the little computer, they would know if they needed to increase the dosage.

"It's my feel-good button," he joked.

That night, Nico's wife, Jodi, gave Jim a jar. On the jar was a label which read, "Papa's Memories." Inside were slips of paper with a memory from each family member, including kids, parents, and siblings. On the back of each slip of paper was written the name of whose memory it was. As we sat around the table together, Jim pulled a paper out of the jar and began reading. His family sitting, or standing, around the table listened intently as Jim read the first one slowly, to himself.

"Dad, you have to read it out loud so we can all hear?" said one of the kids.

"Oh, sorry," he said, with a smile and droopy eyes, as he sat in the wheelchair at the head of the dining room table. He read it aloud. Smiling, he searched the kids' faces, trying to find the person he just guessed was the author of the memory.

"Pick another, Dad!" Which he did. But as he read, his speech was starting to slur. Sitting beside him, I slipped my hand onto his knee as encouragement. We all had to laugh at this memory too. The kids talked on as they remembered that memory also. After a few minutes, their attention went back to their dad. He was holding his head up with his hand, while his elbow rested on the table. In his other hand lay another memory, having already pulled out the next paper, but his eyes were closed. The kids got his attention, wanting him to read more. He tried, but he just couldn't focus.

"Would you like me to read it?" I asked, leaning in close against his side.

"Mm-hm," he said, resting his head against mine for just a minute. I read it, and the kids tried to guess whose it was.

Seeing that he was past tired, I leaned over and asked if he was going to give me the sign. The corner of his lips went up a tired fraction. He tried to pry open his eyes while he shook his head, no. I read a few more, but we could all see that Dad had had a full day. So we decided that it was time for Dad to go to bed.

"Where are you all going?" he asked, trying to hold his eyelids open. "Don't go home on my account."

"It's okay, Dad. You go to bed, we will all be back in the morning," they assured him.

"Okay then. If you insist," he said, with a drooping smile, as I pulled the wheelchair away from the table to get him ready for bed.

That night, after I tucked him in bed, he said he felt alone. He didn't feel God was with him. I assured him He was.

"How can you be sure?" he asked. Going around the bed to climb in on my side, warming him, I asked him to try something with me.

"What?"

"Just close your eyes and trust me."

"Okay, I trust you," he said, closing his eyes with trust in his voice. I prayed silently that God would show Himself to Jim, as he needed Him now.

"Okay, think of your favourite place in the world," I whispered, snuggling up beside him. "Where are you?"

"The beach."

"Look around you. What do you see?" I said, still silently praying for God to show Himself to Jim, as He had to me so many years earlier.

"Water. Sand." he quietly answered.

"Do you see anything else?" I asked, now begging God to show Himself.

"No." Maybe it was too much to ask. A thought entered my mind: *Tell him to turn around.*

"Turn around. What do you see?" I asked in a breathless whisper.

He was quiet. Finally saying in a whisper, "How did you know?" with tears in his voice. We lay there in the darkness, hand in hand, slowly, quietly falling into a peaceful sleep.

People Everywhere

EARLY THE NEXT morning, Jim awoke and wanted to have a shower before anyone else was up. We knew he wouldn't be able to have one as he had in the past. He couldn't stand that long, and our shower stall was way too small to sit on a bench in there. After some thought, we decided to put the shower stool in the tub so he could sit higher, knowing he wouldn't have the strength to get down into the tub. I would use the old rubber shower handle and hose him down.

When Desiree woke up a little later that morning, she heard lots of ruckus coming from the bathroom. Leaning against the door, she asked, "Everyone okay in there? Do you need any help?"

"You do *not* want to come in here," Jim said, and we both started laughing.

"Probably not, but if you need me, I'm out here," she said shyly.

With Jim finally clean, dressed, and shivering, he was back in his wheelchair, resting. After Jim caught his breath, I pushed his wheelchair out into the dining room and left him to talk with Desiree. Then I cleaned up the water that seemed to be everywhere in the bathroom, including on myself. After tidying up, I went to change into something dry. With that out of the way, I started on a few chores as the kids were getting up for breakfast. After a while, Jim asked if I could help him onto the couch so he could sit more comfortably. He thought maybe he could lie down for a bit before his brother Jonathan came to visit. The move from the wheelchair to the couch took his breath away. Shortly he regained some of his strength and went to lay on his right side on the couch.

"Bad idea. Help me up," he said. "I guess laying on that side doesn't work any-more," he added once up. He sat there, trying to concentrate on his breathing. I offered to get a nose/mouth mask for more oxygen. He nodded. I struggled with the super long tubes while trying to exchange his under-the-nose oxygen prongs for a full mask. Even with one of the girls helping, the tubes kept getting all tangled up. My miscalculation with the tubes brought panic to his eyes, as now he had no oxygen. I apologized while finally connecting the proper tube, but he was still stressed. As the kids milled around quietly, I messaged Andrea. She told me to get an Ativan pill from the Symptom Response Kit (SRK) and put it under his tongue to relax him. He soon improved. I hovered, wondering if he was going to be okay.

Meanwhile, his brother Jonathan and his family walked in on this scene. As Jim's oxygen improved, he was able to interact with his brother and family and have a short visit. They then made their way to Mom and Dad's to stay with Dad so Jim's oldest sister Julia could come with Mom. As they left, Nathan came with his family. Nathan and his son Darius sat beside Jim for a bit, having a chat. But when Nathan was dragged away to help Darius find some toys in the other room, Jim motioned for me to come sit beside him.

"I need you. Stay close," he said for my ears only. Turning to Jessica, Nathan's wife, Jim asked, "Jessica would you be able to sing a song at my funeral?" Jim and I had discussed this, she had a beautiful voice, having had many years of vocal lessons.

"Sure, if you want me to," she said, a little surprised.

"But if it is too hard, you may say no," I told her.

Nathan, having re-entered the room, said, "They are taught to sing under pressure. She can do it. She sang at her grandparents' funerals."

Jessica asked Jim, "What song would you like me to sing?"

"I Love to Tell the Story." He requested.

"Do you have any music for that?" she asked, turning to me. I got up and pulled a psalter hymnal off the bookshelf. Finding the song, I handed the open book to Jessica. Looking at the notes on the page, she hummed it while Jim looked on. After a few minutes, she looked up at Jim across the room and said with a smile that she could do this song. Jim smiled, resting back against the couch. A few minutes later, he asked if I could help him to his chair.

"Are you sure?" I asked.

"I need to put my feet up," he said, with a nod of his head. I got the wheelchair ready, but he brushed it aside, feeling he could walk the short distance to the end of the couch where his chair was. With Desiree and I each on a side, we guided him to his chair, where his oxygen dropped again. We decided to change out the oxygen mask to the light green one, the best one, while he relaxed again.

"Just breathe. In, out," I encouraged, holding his hands, crouched on my knees on the floor before him. He sat looking at me while concentrating on his breathing. I smiled at him; he gave a weak smile back. I could see he was exhausted as the lack of oxygen took its toll.

There he sat, in his recliner with an oxygen mask on, as people started to arrive. Besides Elly, Melissa, Calvin, and Josh, who were living here, Desiree and Victoria had stayed the night and were now doing their own things. Nathan, Jessica, and their two kids, Darius and Aria, were joined by Derek, and Danielle with their children Chloe and Parker. Not far behind were Nico and Jodi with their kids, Allie and Graham. They all visited and helped keep the coffee and food going, but had moved to the background so to let the others come in to visit.

I had pulled up a wooden dining room chair beside Jim to be close if he needed anything. Jim's Uncle Rob arrived with his wife, Annette, a dear friend of Jim's before she became his aunt, bringing Mentos peppermints to remind him of years gone by. Our dear friends, Ed and Jennifer, arrived, as well as my brother James, his wife Jane, and their boys, Isaac, Seth, Ethan, and Jayden. Jim, who wanted to be part of the conversation, kept pulling his mask off to talk. Each of these guests came thinking they would be the only ones with Jim. We could visibly see the surprise registering as they entered the full room.

I leaned closer to him after a while and asked him to give me the sign. He shook his head no. At one point, he asked to switch to the other oxygen mask as it was not as noisy as the present one. This one made a soft rushing wind noise that hindered his ability to hear half of what was happening. So we switched them.

A while later, I went to the kitchen, and Desiree took my seat beside him. I just needed to step away. There were so many people. He was so stubborn. I just needed to breathe. In the kitchen, I started busying myself by tidying up. I needed some mindless chore to do—just something, anything, to keep me moving.

I was talking with Annette when Desiree approached us, "Sorry to interrupt, but Dad wants you, Mom." I hurried over to him.

"What's the matter? What do you need?" I asked, crouching in front of him, hoping he would give me the sign.

"I need you. Don't leave me," his voice pleaded from behind the mask as he reached for my hand. "I couldn't see you."

"Sorry. I was just talking in the kitchen," I answered feebly.

Jim's oldest sister arrived with his mom. The people in the room parted to make room for his mom to sit on Jim's right as another dining room chair was set out for her. Quietly coming across the room as the sea of people parted, she sat down. As she turned to him, she reached for his hand, as he reached for hers. Tears welled in my eyes for her. How hard it must be to watch your child go through this.

Jay, the father of one of Jim's recent cadets, arrived, also shocked at the number of people in the room. He found a seat close to Jim and me. A few days ago, I had asked on the church's Facebook page if someone could put Jim's Promise Keepers cassette tape onto a CD for us. Jay was here to pick up the cassette tape and would find a way to do that for us. My brother, overhearing the conversation, asked if it was on Spotify. He looked it up and they found it. Listening to it later, we realized the Spotify version only had the songs, not the Bible verses and words of encouragement that were interspersed between songs.

Then in walked our neighbour Nick.

"Wow! This is a house full!" he exclaimed, looking for Jim. When Nick saw him in his chair across the room, Jim raised his hand and called, "Nick!"

"Hey, Jim. I came to play a game of Rummikub with you, but I see you are busy," he said with a laugh. "I'll come back tomorrow."

"You might not get another chance," Jim said. But Nick, not believing this to be true, prepared to leave. Jim nodded and waved his hand. Jay said his goodbyes, promising to see what he could do as he left with the cassette and Nick.

A bit later, Jim squeezed my hand, motioning for the oxygen reader for his finger. We put it on. His oxygen was reading at 54 percent. I looked at his mom, who was peering down at it too. She looked up at me in shock, reflecting my feelings. I asked him to give me the sign. He shook his head no. I was starting to panic. I felt that if these people would leave, we could get him to relax and increase his oxygen levels. He concentrated on breathing, tried to relax, and got it up to 65 percent. I texted Andrea. "Is the oxygen up to ten? Give him a bolus too," she texted back. I told her we had it at ten, and I was giving him another half tab under his tongue. She double-checked that he was wearing the mask, not the prongs, as his levels climbed to 74 percent with his heart rate at 101. With deep breaths, he was able to get it to 81 percent and started feeling much better.

About an hour and a half later, he was back down between 65 and 70 percent. The struggle was very real, even as he kept pushing his happy button, amid the chatter in the room. Quietly messaging Andrea again, she permitted me to give him another pill under his tongue to relax him. She also asked for the number of the oxygen place to see if there was anything else that they could help us with. "Do you have a lot of people there now?" she asked me, remembering our earlier conversation. Meanwhile, I was texting her that his oxygen level was at 61 percent, and he was really working hard to breathe. His heart rate was now at 139. She told me to give him another Ativan and another bolus (morphine). I pushed his morphine pump button again, not that I felt it would do any good, as he had been pushing it a lot already.

A few minutes later, my phone rang. It was Dr. Thomas. When we told him that Jim still had the oxygen sensor on, he instructed us to take it off. It was probably causing some anxiety.

Not long after that, Jim mumbled something from behind his mask. I leaned in as he repeated that he had to go pee. I wanted to shout, "Thank you, Lord!!"

"Okay, everyone, I need you all to leave the room. Can you please all go to the other room?" After everyone left, I helped him try to pee into the portable urinal. This was not working, so he leaned back in his chair, in the now-empty room, trying to get some rest. I watched him, numb, not knowing what to do. His mom, still beside him, quietly asked how the day went before she arrived. We talked in whispered tones, while our glances kept going to Jim, who sat so still and quiet in his chair. He was trying to say something again while his eyes stayed closed. I got in closer as he repeated that he thought he needed the catheter now. I texted Andrea, and she said she was on her way.

"While we wait, I want to pray with everyone," he requested behind his mask.

"With just the kids?" I asked, not really understanding.

"No, with everyone."

"You want everyone to come back in here and pray together?" I asked with mixed emotions. I had just cleared the room, and now he wanted everyone back in. But his wish was my command. So, I got up, leaving him with his mom, and went to the living room, where everyone milled about visiting.

As I got everyone's attention, I explained, "Jim would like to pray with everyone. Can you please all come back to the other room?" Someone hugged me, but I was not aware of who. Someone else squeezed my arm, but I didn't know who; my brain was in a fog. We returned to the dining room as a hush came over the crowd. People moved around, making room for those still coming. Seeing Desiree and Elly sitting at his feet, he smiled at them. They gave shaky smiles back as tears filled their eyes. He said something to Desiree, and she looked at me for clarification.

"What was that?" I asked, moving closer to him, after shrugging at Desiree.

"Do roll call," he said again, still looking at Desiree.

"Roll call?" we both asked him, and he nodded. I then realized he wanted to know where all his kids were in the sea of people. So, Desiree started calling out the kids' names from oldest to youngest.

"Derek?"

"Here"

"Desiree? Here," she said as everyone snickered.

"Nicolas?" "Here"

"Nathan?" "Here"

"Victoria?" "Here" The single voices came from all over the room.

"Christina?"

"Christina is on her way from Whitby. She will be here soon." We reassured him.

"Elly?" "Here," came the voice at my feet.

"Melissa?" "Here," from somewhere in the back of the room.

"Calvin?" "Here."

"Joshua?" "Here." I looked up to find my thirteen-year-old baby boy close to the door. He was too young to be going through this. As I spied him, I noticed he was not alone. Beside him stood his best friend Lucas, Nick's son. We always joked that Lucas was one of ours as he spent so much time here.

"Lucas?" I said with a smile, continuing the roll call.

"Here!" he said as more snickers broke out in the quiet room, along with Jim's.

"Jim would like us to pray. I'll start, and if anyone wants to pray, they are welcome to," I informed everyone. I prayed with strangled words; I do not remember what I prayed for. Sitting at Jim's feet, my daughter Desiree prayed next, through deeply felt emotion. I remember Jim's sister Julia praying, as well as my brother James. A few others prayed, too, but it was a blur in the midst of sniffles and small sobs. I remember trying to calm myself to finish the prayer after the silence, when Jim started to speak.

"Thank you, Lord, for family and friends. Please be with my family. They are in your hands. I was never the one to care for them. You were. I give them all to you. Amen." I knew he was ready. He had given his life and family over to God. Through my tears, I looked up at the sea of people. Then, I spied Andrea, wondering when she had snuck in. She was making her way to Jim, by way of the outside of the room.

"Dad, Andrew is on the phone. He wants to pray for you," Desiree said as she held out her phone with the speaker on. The few people sitting close around Jim listened as six-year-old Andrew prayed for his Papa. I looked at Desiree, her face showing all her emotion, listening to her precious son pray for her dear father.

Once the call was finished, Andrea had succeeded in making her way beside us. She talked to us for a minute. We decided to move Jim to our bed just around the corner. With no energy left to walk, Jim waited in his chair as we rounded up the older boys. Derek on his right, Nico on his left. These two big boys made a chair around him with their arms. Nathan followed with the morphine pump and had the job of keeping the oxygen tube from kinking on the way to his bed. Trying to lift him up together with minimal jostling, they got into a standing position with Dad in the middle. They took a few steps before Derek said with a strained look, "Dad, I thought you said you lost weight?"

Not missing a beat, Jim replied from behind his oxygen mask, "Sorry. It must have been that last piece of pie!" Those around him burst out laughing, which caused others to wonder what was said. Once his words were repeated for those who hadn't heard, a second round of laughter erupted. I ran ahead to make sure the bed was in a comfortable, slightly elevated position. The boys maneuvered through the short hall and into the bedroom, gently placing their dad on the bed. Once he was comfortable, the boys left so Andrea could put the catheter in. Afterward he lay there, resting for a bit, breathing deeply while listening to loud muffled voices on the other side of the door. I sat on the edge of the bed holding his hand while getting the last instructions from Andrea. I felt like I could finally take a deep breath. I was in my happy place, alone, with the man I love.

Blessed

OPENING HIS EYES a few minutes later, he looked at me, "I want to talk to each of the kids." I sighed.

"You need to rest to get your oxygen levels up."

"I want to talk to each of the kids," he repeated, looking straight at me—that look.

"Each one separately?" I asked, after another sigh. He nodded as he closed his eyes. I went to the kitchen, where some of the kids stood around talking. I told them that Dad wanted to talk to each of them separately. Seeing that Derek was not there, I asked Desiree to sit with Dad while someone went to look for Derek. We brought a dining room chair in, setting it beside Jim. Letting Desiree sit there, I went around to the other side of the bed. Sitting in the middle of my bed, making myself available if he needed anything. Desiree reached for his hand, and he startled awake.

"Oh, sorry, Desiree. Did I fall asleep?" he said after slowly looking at her and registering who it was. She reassured him that it was okay for him to have a nap as no one was going anywhere. Slowly he talked, taking breaks to catch his breath. He gave her some marriage advice. Then had some funny quip for her. Lastly, he asked her if she had any questions for him, or if there was anything she needed to say. After I love you's, she left the room and got Derek.

Derek came in and sat down on the chair beside his dad. "Hey, Dad!" he said confidently, taking Jim's hand. Jim opened his eyes and turned his head to see his oldest. He gave the same marriage advice. Then he closed his eyes for a minute, taking some deep breaths. After a few breaths, he continued with a funny quip and then asked Derek if he had anything he wanted to ask. "Cause now's the time," he said.

Nico and Nathan also got the same marriage advice, but it was harder now. He would start, but he was tiring, taking more breaks. Finally, looking at me, "You tell them." So, I would tell them what he told the others.

"Is that right?" I asked him, and he nodded his agreement. Then he would say something that pertained to each of them personally. Finally, he would finish with, "Ask me whatever you need to ask me now."

In the kitchen, the kids waited their turns. As one came out, they all wanted to hear what Dad said that was funny, and they each had something. Next, Victoria went in with her boyfriend, Seth. Then Christina, who had returned from Whitby, went in with her husband, Cody—followed by Elly and later Melissa. Jim was taking more breaks in between now. His energy was fully spent, but he pushed on as he ran this race. I went to get Calvin and Josh, but neither of them wanted to go in, not wanting to see their dad like this.

"I understand, but Dad wants to talk to you. Just step in the doorway so you can hear what he says." My heart hurt for them, but I didn't want them to regret not going to see him, to listen to what Jim had to say to them, to be blessed by him.

Finally, I got Calvin to come with me. He stood beside me and the bed.

"Jim, Calvin's here," I said, and his eyes slowly fluttered open. Jim held out his hand and took Calvin's. He told him he loved him and to be good for his mom. After a few more words and tears all around, Calvin left, with me behind him in search of Josh.

"Dad and I have talked already," Josh pointed out once I found him hanging out in the other room. "I really don't want to go in there," he stressed again.

"Dad is just lying in bed like he always does. He has on his oxygen mask," I explained, hoping to make it easier for him. "I will stand right beside you and hold your hand if you like," I suggested, hoping this would change his mind. Finally, he reluctantly followed me, not knowing what to expect. Standing just inside the silent room, we watched Jim sleep as I let Joshua orient himself. As Jim's eyelids fluttered open, he looked at Joshua and, rallying his strength, softly said he was sorry that he couldn't be there for him as he grew up. Joshua started to cry, and I pulled him into a hug with me between him and Jim. We stood there in each other's arms, crying. Jim was too exhausted to say anything more, so he closed his eyes. After a few long minutes, Joshua shifted a bit and started to shake as more sobs came from deep down. After a few minutes of trying to console him, I turned to look at Jim. It was only then that I noticed Jim was holding Joshua's hand and lovingly looking at him with tears in his eyes as well. I knew that no words were necessary. The love and encouragement that was shared between those hands and eyes would go on in Joshua's heart for his lifetime.

Think about it.

Have you blessed your children? Jacob's blessing of his twelve sons on his deathbed in Genesis 48 and 49 is a great model. Blessings are meant to be a guide for the future. Jacob's model even shows how to bless those who fall short and have lived a less-than-godly life. A kind word can be a blessing. God gave us the power to heal others, and in the process, this heals us. Make a difference and bless your children today.

"The Lord your God has blessed you in all the work of your hands" (Deuteronomy 2:7).

Around 8:00 that evening, after resting for a bit, Jim announced he had to go to the bathroom. I reminded him that he had the catheter in, but he shook his head and said he needed to go number two. Now, how on earth were we going to do this? I texted Andrea for words of wisdom. I walked into the kitchen deep in thought, not knowing what to do. I stood there staring. Noticing I was deep in thought, some of the girls asked what was wrong. I told them that Dad needed to go to the bathroom, and I had no idea how to make that work for him. Going back into the bedroom, Jim suggested a plan. Collecting a five-gallon pail, we set it beside the bed. On top of it, we set the handicapped toilet riser. Perfect, our own homemade commode. With some help Jim was able to do his business, and we got him comfortably back in bed again. Andrea texted asking how the transfer went when I explained what we had done. I texted back, "Lol. His idea... see, I still need him. He did better than I thought he would."

Once he was sleeping peacefully, I headed into the living room where the kids were hanging out, not even registering that the guests had all left. As I entered, they all came around me. "How is he?"

"He is resting." Knowing that they wanted to know what to expect, I continued, "I don't know what to expect, guys. We just have to go one day at a time. Thanks for being here."

"We wouldn't want to be anywhere else, Mom," someone said.

"What are your plans now?" I asked, looking around. The boys said they would bring their wives home and help tuck the kids into bed, but they were coming back. Christina and her husband would be staying too.

"Mom, we are all staying," someone said, as tears filled my eyes.

"Thanks, guys, I'm going to go to bed now. I'm exhausted. I'll leave the door open, and you guys can come to sit beside Dad anytime you want. We should probably make sure someone is always with him. But I'm going to sleep now." I didn't want them to feel pushed away. If they needed to be there, I wanted to make that available. I knew that's what Jim would have wanted too.

When I returned to the bedroom after preparing for bed, Jim was sleeping soundly. Curling up beside him, my face contorted, and my body shook with the pain of losing my best friend, the love of my life. I was starting to think this would probably be the last night I had with him. I forced myself not to worry about the future, but to love him this minute, and every minute I still had with him. Sobbing, I fell into a restless sleep.

Jim, woke at the same time as every other morning, but with a little bit of a hazy mind. With a startled look, he looked over to the end of the bed where three of our daughters sat.

"What are you girls doing in my room?" he asked.

"Just hanging out, Dad. Making sure you're okay," they said.

I think we were all somewhat shocked that he was as alert as he was, I snuggled in closer as he wrapped his arm around me. The girls got up and left saying, "Eew, yuk!" and "Do you have to?" as we smiled at each other. I didn't stay there long before I felt I needed to drag myself out of bed before Andrea arrived.

Jan messaged, "Good morning, brother? How are you this morning?" I saw it later, having forgotten about Jim's morning ritual. I messaged back, "Sorry, Jim cannot message you anymore, Jan. How are you?" From then on, I promised myself I would message Jan in the mornings with an update as long as Jim was here.

This morning Jim continued asking what time it was. I figured he didn't want to miss the 9:00 am church service. But the time was to spring ahead one hour, and the nurse was to come at 9:00. I made the decision not to change the clocks and let him think the nurse was there at 8:00 and we would watch online after she left, telling everyone my plan.

As the nurse worked with Jim, I left for a few minutes to let the kids know that I would watch church with Dad in the bedroom on the laptop, and they could watch on the big TV screen in the dining room. But they informed me they were all coming into our room to watch church with Dad.

"How are you all going to fit in there? How do you plan on doing that?" I questioned. But I wasn't against the idea.

"Leave it to us, Mom. We will figure it out," they assured me. And they did. Putting a cookie sheet on the shelf in my closet with weight on the back, they had the laptop hanging out of the closet. Derek connected his blue tooth speaker so everyone could hear it. Rearranging furniture, they brought stools for the back row and chairs for the sides. Others climbed into my bed, propping their backs against the wall, while someone else used their legs as a backrest. All ten children (and one son-in-law and a grandbaby) were there, surrounding their dad, who lay sleeping in his bed. We started the service, all joining in the song for the call to worship, "Restore My Soul."[12]

As we started singing, Jim's eyes flew open, startled by the voices that surrounded him. As he took in all of his children, his eyes opened wider, and his smile grew bigger and bigger. I sat in the corner watching him, as tears streamed down my cheeks. A dream had come true for both of us this morning, one we had prayed for and wondered if it would ever happen in our lifetime. Our children were all worshiping with us, worshipping God Almighty, creator of all! Jim looked at me with the biggest smile and started to sway to the music. He was a happy man as he worshiped God with that big smile on his face. After the song, he lay back and settled in for the service, again looking at everyone around him. But he didn't have the strength to stay awake, and he fell asleep again.

As Pastor Martin began reading the passage for today's sermon, Jim woke again. He motioned for his water and Desiree helped him get a sip from his water bottle straw. Before replacing his oxygen mask, he looked up at the screen as Pastor Martin was finishing the reading.

"Sorry, Pastor, I think I missed that. Could you repeat that for me?" Jim said for everyone in the crowded room to hear.

"He's only reading it once, Dad!" Nathan said as a burst of laughter rang out from all of those around. We were all remembering the words Jim would regularly say before reading devotions at the dinner table in the evenings.

"Listen up, for I'm only going to read this once," he would say.

As the service was coming to a close, Parker, Derek's son, came running into the house. He was expecting to see lots of people, but the house was quiet and no one was milling about. Coming to the open bedroom door and seeing everyone inside, he came to a sudden stop at the doorway.

"What are you guys all doing in there?" he said with a puzzled look on his three-year-old face. We all laughed as we got up to give Papa some time to rest.

---

[12] Andi Rozier, "Restore My Soul," All Essential Music, 2006.

Since it was still the weekend, more people came and went as Jim had request-ed. But now he stayed in bed and slept through most of those visits, only waking occasionally, each time surprised to see someone in his room. I found myself hov-ering in the hall as others sat with him. I watched for signs of stress so I could push his morphine pump. When he woke, I would have to talk to him, asking him to keep the oxygen mask on even though he wanted to talk to those around him. If he took it off, even for a few minutes, he would struggle for air. I was also concerned about him getting bed sores. At one point, I asked him how his bum was.

"My bum is fine. How's yours?" he asked with a twinkle in his eye and a mischie-vous smile on his lips as he raised his eyebrows.

"Jim!" I said, blushing in shock, not knowing who would be listening. He chuckled.

Neighbours, homeschooling friends, and members of our church family were call-ing and bringing huge meals—including a breakfast one morning—to feed all of us who were here. Having taken over my kitchen, the girls were struggling to find room in the fridge for leftovers. Meanwhile, the kitchen island had snacks ready for any time of the day, as well as Derek's old Nintendo, a game from years gone by. The younger boys were learning all the tricks of the game, while still trying to wrap their heads around losing everything if they walked away from the game. Through the large archway off the kitchen was the dining room, where the big screen TV had Wii set up. Melissa's big screen TV had been brought down from upstairs to play Xbox at the end of the room. On the dining room table was a large Jan Van Haasteren puzzle that Jan and Wilma had given us. The furniture in the room was all moved to accommodate these activities. At any given time, you might find someone under a pile of quilts or blankets on the couch or a mattress that had also been brought down from the girl's room, trying to get a little bit of sleep. The only way to tell if it was night or day was the amount of light that shone in through the four extra-large windows and eight-foot patio door. Or if you heard small children running the hall outside our bedroom, no one telling them to be quiet because we all knew Papa loved a house with little running feet. The children's laughter and squeals could be heard all day as they were so excited to be playing with their cousins. At one point, Jim's mom commented on the noise. We told her that it was the way Jim wanted it. Our kids, when not taking turns with their dad, would be gaming, puzzling, or playing a card game with boisterous voices.

Jim awoke at one point and looked at me. "They are having fun!" he said with a huge smile.

"Yes. They are playing games," I said.

"They are playing Wizard!" he said, closing his eyes again with a smile firmly in place. I knew his mind was back to the summer at the cottage with his five boys for their treasured "Dad and the Lad's" weekend.

By late Sunday, the kids realized that they didn't want to leave. I listened as the older boys discussed not going to work next week. Nico smiled and let the other two know he took off this week a few weeks ago. He had already asked me for Dad's garage to-do list and would start on it Monday morning. Derek and Nathan contacted their bosses and let them know what was going on and that they would probably not be in next week. It was around that time that I realized that the kids were all home, really home, and they were planning on staying even though I didn't ask them to. My heart swelled with love and emotion.

Humour and Heaven

I THINK IT was Monday. Jim was still in his bed, with his younger sister Mary holding his left hand while sitting on my side of the bed. His older sister Julia sat in a chair, holding his right hand. As I stood in the doorway, I couldn't believe that his sisters were talking and arguing as these sisters do. "Now of all the times?" I wondered to myself. But then I noticed Jim's eyes open, and he nodded to Mary for his water. He pulled down his oxygen mask as she reached for the water bringing it to his lips. He took a sip from the straw, sloshing it around in his mouth. Turning to Julia, he sprayed that water out from between his teeth. Making an arch which fell short, landing on her lap. He wiped his mouth, replaced the mask, laid back and closed his eyes. We all sat there stunned for a minute before bursting out in laughter.

"Oh, Jim! I knew you always loved me best. Thanks for always looking out for me," said Mary, the dry sister.

"Well!" said Julia with mocked shock.

I was shocked, and yet my heart warmed, feeling light. Even though he was no longer talking, he was still getting his point across in a humourous way that only he could do.

Julia and her husband Henk had offered to be on call whenever Jim's Mom needed to come. I was getting ready for bed that night when Julia called and asked if they could come, as Mom wanted to sit with Jim for a bit even though it was so late. How could I say no, hoping my kids would allow me that same privilege if I was in that position? Julia dropped her husband off to sit with Dad and came with Mom. Jim's younger brother, Jonathan, came from London, meeting them here at around midnight. Letting Mom and Jonathan sit with Jim while he slept, Julia hung out in the kitchen in the next room. Here she watched as my boys rummaged through the kitchen looking for food to eat. Finding nothing that was quick and of the "junk food" category, they claimed there was nothing to eat. Julia texted her sister Mary to tell her we had no food in the house and the following day Mary arrived with fruit trays and buns—leaving my daughters with the challenge of finding more room in the fridge.

At one point, a new nurse, Dorie, came to the house as it was Andrea's weekend off. I led Dorie to our room, stepping aside to allow her to enter. She stopped in the doorway.

"He looks so healthy considering he has cancer," she said in shock as she looked at Jim lying in the bed. I tried to look at him through her eyes. He was not a frail man at all. His face was somewhat full, yet his cheekbones were more pronounced. His eyes were not sunk in. His arms that lay on top of the sheet still had muscle on them. He had been up and fully participating in life less than two weeks ago. It was good to see him through her eyes before I turned to get the Symptom Response Kit for her.

"You can use the island in the kitchen if you would like more room," I said, re-entering the room to see her spreading stuff out on my side of the bed.

"No, I like to work close to the patient to observe them," she said as we talked about Jim and how he had been doing.

"He gets restless and starts to groan, louder at times, so I push his morphine button," I said as she was putting together some syringes with medication that I would need to give Jim. I was getting nervous; I didn't feel qualified to do that. She explained that I was to give him a syringe of Nozinan in the port they had in his stomach every hour as needed to help with restlessness. There was also midazolam, a sedative I was to give him every two hours as needed that would put him out like if he was in surgery. Jim moaned louder.

"It's okay, Jim, we are not giving that to you now," she reassured him as she continued to work. "Have you noticed that he is responding to you," she asked me. I shook my head no. "He thinks he is talking and that you can understand what he is saying. Like now he is upset about the medication we are talking about," she informed me. I looked over at Jim as this suddenly made sense to me. He was not restless earlier; he was telling me something. I wished I had known that sooner. Dorie encouraged me to talk to the kids and ask if anyone wanted to be with Dad at the end. If so, then they needed to stay close, as he could leave us in a few hours or a few days.

Once the medication was all prepared and labelled for me, Dorie moved around the bed to stand beside Jim. She checked the sight of the morphine pump and explained that as the morphine collects under the skin it makes a hard lump and is no longer easily absorbed. Therefore, she needed to change the location of the pump site on his belly. We called Nathan, the closest at hand, to come in and hold Dad's legs down while I had his hands. His eyes flew open as stomach hair came off with the tape, and he groaned loudly while Dorie apologized. I offered to get the shaver to shave the new location for the next one so it wouldn't be so painful when we needed to move it again. Jim groaned in agreement. Once I had shaved a spot clear on his stomach and the new morphine line was in, she placed a pick line in for me to administer the new meds. As she repacked the Symptom Response Kit and put the garbage away, Dorie assured me she would return and said if I needed anything, just to give her a call.

A few hours later, while Victoria and her boyfriend Seth were sitting on chairs beside Jim, he started to get restless. Taking a deep breath, I looked in the little brown notebook to see what I was supposed to do. Climbing onto my side of the bed with a disinfectant wipe and a syringe, I took another deep breath while Victoria and Seth looked on.

"Are you okay, Mom?" Victoria asked.

"No. 'Give as needed,' they say. How am I supposed to know when that is, what that looks like?" I said this as tears filled my eyes. Swiping them away, I tried to concentrate, remembering what Dorie had told me. Unscrewing the end of the port, I cleaned it off. Screwing on the syringe, I slowly, very slowly pushed down the plunger. When it was completely down, I unscrewed it from the port and set it aside, screwing on the cap. A sob broke through as I finished. More were quick to follow as I rested my head on his chest, and my body went limp beside him. Victoria and Seth quietly left, closing the door behind them to give me my space.

"Lord, why? I can't do this anymore. It hurts too much to see him like this. I am so not qualified to give him these meds. Please, Lord, take him home. Take him to you." Wondering how much longer this would go on, I lay there till the sobs subsided. My days were becoming blurred, but God was reminding me to endure. To trust in Him in the midst of so much discouragement. Something in my soul bowed before that invitation. I would climb out of our bed and be brave. I would overcome the weight of the burden before me.

Monday was March 14, Pi (3.14) Day. Later that day Desiree told me we had received a total of ten pies from different people in two hours! She didn't know what to do with them all. After some discussion, we decided that we would put them in the freezer and take them out for the funeral since that was Dad's favourite dessert. Except for the lemon pies, which the boys were happy to help devour.

Upon my request, the kids started going through the photo albums and scanning photos, while others looked through photos stored on USB sticks, trying to find photos for the funeral. The older kids related to the younger ones what it was like when they were younger living with Dad. They shared and laughed about many stories.

I spent a lot of time hanging out at the door frame those days looking in as others hung out in my bedroom. The place which used to be our sanctuary, a place to get away from the everyday—our place. If you asked me where my favourite place in the world was two years earlier, or even a month earlier, I would have told you, my bedroom. With a large family and everyone always vying for my and Jim's attention, we needed a place that was just ours—a haven. My haven was now being filled with other bodies, but also with a whole lot of prayer. God was here. I could feel it.

We made sure someone was always with Jim as he lay in bed, either lying on my side of the bed or sitting beside him on the chair while holding his hand. It was heartbreaking watching my daughters curl up beside their daddy and weep. Weep for the times they would still need their dad. Weep for the time Dad wouldn't be there to walk them down the aisle or to hold their newborn babies. For the time he would have taught his grandsons that John Deere makes the best tractors ever. But mostly just to be the godly father and Papa they still needed each and every day.

It was beautiful watching my older sons hold their dad's hand and promise to care for those he would leave behind. And yet I knew they would miss his advice, guidance, and humour. My heart hurt watching the two youngest hover outside the door, steeling glances inside at their Dad, seeing the confusion and loss on their faces.

Calvin said he really wanted to say something at Dad's funeral, so I encouraged him to write it down. When he was done, he admitted he didn't think he would be able to say it in front of everyone. I encouraged him to say it to Dad because that's really all that mattered. So, he stepped just inside the room and closed the door. Hesitating, he looked at me.

"It's okay. Dad can hear you, Calvin, even if he doesn't open his eyes or say anything." He spoke special heartfelt words to his dad and I videotaped the scene that unfolded in front of me for him to watch years from now.

The kids wanted us to have time together, too, so they respected our privacy when I would close the door. This is when I would read our devotions to him and pray with him, when I would weep beside him or on his chest. I would whisper in his ear about the special times that were just ours, memories that only we shared. Then I would reassure him that we would be okay. God had us in his hands.

During one of my quiet times with Jim, having finished our devotions, I told him we needed a nap because I was so tired. Snuggling up close to him, I fell into an exhausted sleep. Suddenly my door flew open, and Desiree stood there mumbling quick apologies followed by, "The hydro is off. Dad's oxygen machine is off!" As she disappeared, she yelled back, "I'm going to tell the boys!" As my brain registered the stillness, an understanding slammed into my brain. I flew out of bed and into the hall. Stopping suddenly just outside my bedroom door, in the middle of the hall, I looked left and right.

"What do I do? What do I do?" I said aloud to myself. Then I heard a click, followed by the loud hum of the oxygen machine to my right and a softer hum of the fridge farther in front of me. As the hum registered, my heart rate started to come down, and my brain made me breathe again. Desiree returned with an exasperated look on her face.

"The boys *accidentally* turned the main breaker off in the garage." With relief, I returned to my spot beside Jim, knowing that he had heard the whole thing.

"Those kids will be the death of us yet!" I said to Jim, to which he groaned in agreement.

Later the boys told me that Desiree returned to the garage where they were working on Nathan's four-wheeler with the younger two boys and gave them an earful.

"What were you guys thinking? That was Dad's oxygen you turned off! And not only that, but I was on the eighth world of Mario Brothers, and now it's all gone!" As her sternness eroded away, the boys said, "Well, we see where your priorities lie," and they all laughed together.

As time passed it got harder and harder for the children to sit with Jim. His breathing was becoming more laboured, and yet he seemed so peaceful. Having not had anything to eat or drink for a few days, his muscles started to get tight. I couldn't move his head straight. His hands started to curl. It looked painful, yet his brow was relaxed.

"Mom, are they not going to give him IV or any fluids?" asked one of the girls with concern.

"It will just prolong the inevitable," I said sadly as realization dawned on her face.

Think about it

Each of us, you and me, needs to be taken to a place where God alone is sufficient. Suffering takes you to that place. No one is exempt from suffering. It is a crucial part of every person's life, moulding us into who we are. But will you turn to God to pull you out of the depths? Will you call to God for your strength? It is your choice. He is waiting.

"So I say to you: Ask and it will be given to you; seek and you will find; knock and the door will be opened to you. For everyone who asks receives; he who seeks finds; and to him who knocks, the door will be opened" (Luke 11:9–10).

Tuesday night, or perhaps the wee hours of Wednesday morning, I awoke and heard the change in his breathing. It sounded more like a coffee percolator. As I opened my eyes, I saw my oldest son holding his dad's hand and rubbing his own eyes with his other hand. These long days were taking a toll on us all. He looked over at me, and I tried to give him a brave smile. Without saying a word, we both knew it would be soon. Silently I sent up a prayer that God would take him home. I whispered to Derek the story of when he came into this world, our first child, a son.

"Dad didn't know I could see him from my hospital bed as he stood in the hall looking inside the nursery window at you. He was crying. I had never seen him cry. Not till more recently have I seen him cry. You made him a dad! He is so proud of you." We continued to share memories in whispered tones. Desiree slipped in about an hour later. She also shared some of the stories that she and Derek, being the oldest, shared. We smiled and giggled as Jim's percolator-breathing continued. After a time, Derek asked Desiree if she was going to stay.

"I can't sleep. I just needed to be here," she said.

"I'm going to try to get a bit of sleep then. Just wake me if anything changes," Derek said. I realized then that he had been there the whole night.

Desiree and I talked a bit more before I laid back down beside the love of my life. With tears in my eyes and a sore jaw from trying to control the tears, I hovered in and out of sleep, listening to Jim's breathing. Slowly I noticed that it was changing again. I forced myself to listen as my eyelids stayed shut.

In, out. In, out...(stillness)

Deep breath in, out. In, out...(stillness)

Deep breath in, out. I was so tired; did I miss it? I opened my eyes to see Desiree crying, and my heart broke for her. She saw me looking at her and tried to put on a brave shaky smile.

In, out... I notice I'm holding my breath in anticipation of his next breath.

Big breath in, out... two, three, four, five. Six.

IN, out... was that his last breath?

IN, out... no, is this it?... We wait. How long do you wait?

"Lord, take him, please." The words don't make it past my lips. Desiree and I look at each other with tear-filled eyes as we realize our silent prayers have been answered. Jim is with his Lord and Saviour.

I feel numb inside, confused. What do I do now?

Desiree quietly gets up, "I'll get Derek," she says as she leaves the room toward where the oxygen machine is still humming loudly in the quiet house. I slowly climbed out of bed from beside my husband of thirty-two years for the last time. In a daze, I rounded the bed and stood at his feet, looking down at him. His eyes, which used to twinkle mischief, are closed, and his head is bent sideways as in sleep. His sunken cheeks make his cheekbones even more prominent. The oxygen mask hid his beautiful lips that would no longer kiss me. I took a second look, a closer look. Jim was not there. I couldn't feel his presence, his warmth. It was only a shell.

"Till we meet again, my love. I'm right behind you," I whispered. And I walked out of the room, closing the door quietly behind me.

Think about it

Our time here on earth is short—a mist that vanishes. Think of a rope that goes on forever, and a small strip of tape is wrapped around the very end to keep it from fraying. The tape represents the time you have here on this earth. The rest of the rope represents eternity. What you do with your time on that tape will determine where you will spend the rest of eternity. Remember to focus on things that truly matter for eternity. Make the most of every moment.

"The world and its desires pass away, but the man who does the will of God lives forever" (1 John 2:17).

Humour Lives On

IN THE KITCHEN, I texted Dorie to let her know that Jim had passed. She called to let me know she would be right over to get Jim ready for the funeral home. I then called Jim's mom. Meanwhile, the kids were all awake now, mulling about in hushed tones. I called my parents and messaged his family and our prayer partners:

"Blessed is everyone who fears the Lord, who walks in his ways." Today my dear, loving husband and best friend went to be with his Lord and Saviour. We were truly blessed to have him in our lives. His sense of humour and practical jokes as well as his witness for the Lord will be truly missed.

I gathered his suit, the one he wore for a few of the kids' weddings, his signature blue shirt and matching tie, along with a t-shirt, underwear, and a pair of socks. Dorie arrived and disconnected all the wires and tubes from Jim's body. Pastor Martin arrived shortly after that to talk with the family. And Jeff and Curtis Lockhart arrived to take away the body. Pastor Martin prayed with us and asked us to share stories as we all looked around at each other, tired.

"We have been sharing so many stories this week," someone finally said.

"I would like to get to know some of them to share as I put together his service," he nudged. That is when the stories, repeated stories, started to surface again. He also asked if anyone would like to say a few words at the funeral.

"I would like to, but I don't know if I will make it through," said Desiree.

"I'll go with you Desiree," said Elly.

"Will you guys all write something funny about dad? Just keep it light 'cause we have to make it through," Desiree requested.

"I can do some too," said Melissa, to everyone's surprise. We agreed that everyone would email Desiree and Elly something to say.

Partway through, Jeff Lockhart came in to inform us they were ready and would be leaving. With Pastor Martin on hand, we took a minute to make plans to have the visitation on Friday and the funeral on Saturday.

"The mask mandate is still in place but is to be lifted on Monday if you wanted to wait until Monday," Jeff suggested.

"No, my kids have taken more than enough time off for us. I want to be considerate and do it before Sunday. That way they can have a quiet day before returning to work," I responded. He then asked if some of us could stop by to go over the final details later that day. Desiree and Elly offered to go with me, and we set a time. As he left, I remembered the shirt Jim had on now. The girls talked about making a memory quilt, and they wanted to use that shirt in the quilt too. Derek being by the door, offered to catch them before they left. Returning a few minutes later, he nodded and said Jeff promised to keep it. A little later, Pastor Martin took his leave also.

The order of everyone else's funeral clothing surfaced. We decided that the older boys would take the younger two to London that afternoon to shop for suits. My three daughters-in-law smiled at me, promising to go along and help the boys as their conversation had turned to camo suits. I mouthed a thank you to them. Next we tried on shoes, making sure they fit. Nico would be wearing Jim's shoes as he needed a pair, and Jim didn't.

The daughters and I agreed to go shopping the next day, Thursday, for new dresses. We would then go for a family dinner out at Pizza Hut, Dad's favourite. Nathan called around, and the only Pizza Hut that had a dine-in due to COVID was in London. As this was in honour of dad, that's where we needed to go.

My friend Jennifer called to give her condolences and ask if there was anything she could do. "Can you please come for a walk with me after I meet with the funeral director? I have so many kinks from sitting on that bed at weird angles," I asked, and she happily agreed. Good friends are treasures during times like these.

Again, the phone rang. This time it was Rene, the best man from our wedding, who lived out west.

"How are you holding up, Joanne?" came the concerned voice.

"I'm okay, Rene. It was a good week. Even if it was a sad time, it was a *good* time," I said with sincerity. He asked a few more questions and had a great listening ear. Then with sadness in his voice, he let me know that he wouldn't be able to make it to the funeral as his wife's uncle's funeral would also be on Friday.

"That is okay Rene. You need to be there for your wife. We can't have the interment until after April. Maybe you can come then?" I asked.

"Oh yes. I'll be there!" He was relieved there was still a second option. Truthfully, so was I. I knew that I would need him here as much as he would need to be here.

Later that day, as I drove to the funeral home, I asked the girls to help me come up with some way to show Dad's personality in the obituary. They were at a loss, as was I.

We were welcomed into the funeral home and sat down in front of Jeff's neat and tidy desk. He went over a few details, confirming what Jim and I had already decided. I confirmed the casket we had picked and how the visitation and funeral would be held at our church in Stratford. We also confirmed that the interment would have to wait until April or later, as the graveyard wouldn't be opening any graves until then. Secretly, we were thankful for this as then it could be a private affair like the kids wanted.

Derek even said later, "It might make it harder, but then we will be out of the fog of these days. It will be more meaningful, but harder."

Then it was time for the obituary. Yes, we wanted a bible verse. I would get Jeff the one Jim had on the table beside his chair: *"Therefore we do not loose heart. Even though our outward man is perishing, yet the inward man is being renewed day by day. For our light affliction, which is but for a moment, is working for us a far more exceeding and eternal weight of glory, while we do not look at the things which are seen, but at the things which are not seen. For the things which are seen are temporary, but the things which are not seen are eternal"* (2 Corinthians 4:16–18). He then went through every line that would be in the obituary. We went through the names of the kids and their spouses and then the grandkids. I was thankful that he already had the correct spelling of everyone's names from the list I had brought him weeks earlier. But when he got to Jim's parents, a lightbulb went off in my head.

"Son of Art and Corrie Schreuders," he said as I looked over at the girls with a sneaky smile. They looked back at me, confused.

"Can we change that to 'Favourite son of Art and Corrie Schreuders'?" I said with a smile.

"Umm, are we going to start World War III with that?" he asked nervously.

The girls' faces lit up and together said, "No, it won't. Yes, Mom, you have to do that!" they giggled, knowing this is what I was looking for when we talked on the way over.

"Okay. If you are sure," he said, still unsure himself.

"Yes, it will be fine," we assured him.

"Favourite son of Art and Corrie Schreuders," he said while he typed it into his computer, and on he continued. Before we left, he handed me twenty death certificate forms in a white envelope to use later. He also said he would email me a copy of the obituary later today to approve before he posted it online and send it out to the newspapers of our choosing. I also asked him about payment, to which he said we could pay for it in the next month or so once the estate had been settled. I was relieved.

Once finished, we walked together across two streets to the florist. Here we were following Jeff's orders to get a casket arrangement that would be delivered to the funeral home. We thought these were expensive—we girls never buy flowers. We bit the bullet and looked for something that would suit us.

"Do you carry oriental lilies?" I asked, thinking of the beautiful flowers that were in our wedding bouquet.

"We can special order them for you," the lady offered. Knowing this would take time, we agreed to do something else. But what? The lady asked what we were looking for.

"We are looking for a casket arrangement for my husband, who passed away," I said for the first time aloud, tears wanting to push to the surface.

Shoving them back down, I heard Desiree ask, "If we bring in a toy John Deere tractor could you build it into the arrangement?"

"Absolutely," said the lady behind the counter with a big smile.

"We will get Nico to pick out a good one from Dad's collection," she said. Well, that takes care of the colouring, I thought. Green and yellow. I paid for the arrangement with the promise to bring the tractor in later that day.

The girls and I giggled on the way home, "What would the family think of what Mom did?" But now I was getting a little nervous. Maybe I shouldn't have done that. Jim was the one who kept my crazy ideas in check. Now I just had me.

As we came to the house, I noticed Jennifer was already waiting for me, visiting with the girls who were still home. With a deep breath, Jennifer and I set out down the road, just the two of us. It felt so good to walk at a brisk pace, stretching all those kinked muscles. As we walked, she listened to me talk about the past days and how beautiful the last week was, even in the midst of sadness. I felt so much better speaking my story and physically moving. I felt I could go on; I felt God's peace.

Think about it

You might want to help a friend or loved one when they have lost someone close to them, but you don't know what to do. You feel helpless as you stand by watching them hurt. The best thing you can do is *listen*. The hurting person needs to process what has happened and especially to talk about the person who is now gone. You can talk about happy memories of their loved one, but let the one hurting do most of the talking. Someday the hurting friend will again ask how you and your family are, but right now, the grief is all-consuming. Yes, there will be tears, but these tears are *very* healing. If you're the one hurting don't apologize for the tears; let them flow.

Back at home, I found the obituary in my email, and I sent it to all the family members with a link to the church website for those who wanted to watch the service online. I then started working on the "Life and Times of Jim Schreuders" bulletin for the funeral. The boys arrived and spread out the clothes they just purchased, as the girls shared what Mom had done on the obituary.

"Way to go, Mom!" they laughed. I noticed a few butterflies in my stomach over this. "Please Lord, help them all see it as the joke it was intended to be." I prayed silently.

Finishing off the bulletin I had some of the kids read over it.

Jim was born August 1, 1967, to Art and Corrie Schreuders of St. Marys, Ontario. He grew up on the family pig farm with his older sister Julia, younger sister Mary, and his younger brother Jonathan. All his life he has been known for his sense of humour and his way of making people feel at ease.

Jim met Joanne during a Stratford-Wellandport youth exchange in the fall of 1987. December of the following year he planned a fancy dinner and limo ride to Niagara Falls. At the falls, where the water falls over the edge, Jim popped the big question, promising Joanne that life with him would always be exciting, never dull. He kept that promise in the thirty-two years of marriage that started in the fall of 1989.

They started their life together in Tavistock, Ontario where Jim worked as an apprentice mechanic for the local New Holland dealer. In 1990 they moved to Georgetown where he enjoyed the semi-retired life as a farm field manager while getting to know his wife better and starting a million-dollar family with a Derek and Desiree.

The beginning of 1993 brought them back to St. Marys where they started working long hours in their own business Western Farm Hand doing relief milking and chores for various farmers in the area. To fill some of the extra hours he worked for Logan Ford in St. Marys as a mechanic. During this time another two sons, Nicolas and Nathan, and two daughters, Victoria and Christina, were added to the growing clan.

Over the years, he was on church counsel and taught Sunday school. But his true love was Cadets. Did you know he had been teaching boys (and even a few years as a head counsellor) since he was sixteen years old?

In 1997 Jim decided to accept a job with Fawcett Tractor Supply in St. Marys as a sales representative. This being an 8–5 job, he looked forward to more time for his growing family. Which only assisted in growing his family by two more daughters, Elizabeth and Melissa. Realizing they needed a larger house, they purchased their first home in Fullarton in 2003. During this time, they leaned on God as Joanne was diagnosed with a tumour at the base of her brain on her spine. God was gracious through that time and allowed them more time together. Another two sons, Calvin and Joshua, joined the family that was really important to Jim. During this time, Jim stayed with Fawcetts for seventeen years. Jim was then offered his "dream job" in 2014 as a farm equipment salesperson for John Deere Premier in Listowel. As time passed, he felt his talents maybe did lie more in the line of parts/sales and accepted a transfer to Premier Tavistock in parts and sales at the beginning of 2020. This transfer also made it possible for him to be close to his parents to help when needed. This transfer we now see as a blessing from God as Jim discovered cancer in his leg during this time. It was the same cancer as Terry Fox. "With new medical advances you get to keep your leg!" he was told. This fast-growing cancer made its way to his lungs and after multiple rounds of radiation and surgery, it finally took on a life of its own.

During all this time Jim clung to the Lord and the Hope we all have in Him. His laughter and teasing NEVER left him. On Saturday, March 12, with a room full of family and friends Jim asked for us to pray. With many tears, we prayed for Jim to have strength as he finished this journey here on earth and he prayed for us who were left behind. Giving us all up to our Lord and Saviour who can do immeasurably more than he ever could. His sons carried him to his room where he was able to talk to each of his children separately. Jim encouraged each of them in their walk, giving them their own funny memory and answering any last questions they might have. Sunday, Joanne and the children crowded around him as they watched church online and sang together while Jim smiled his big smile, swaying to the music. As Jim requested, family and friends continued to come (a big revolving door) sitting, visiting, and enjoying each other's company.

Wednesday, March 16, around 7:00 am Jim took his last breath and entered into glory. Jim said from the beginning that he wanted to do this well. Time and again we have all seen him do this well. To God give the Glory! AMEN and AMEN!

Later that evening I found a message from Jim's younger brother Jonathan, "'Favourite son of Art and Corrie Schreuders.' Jimmy's idea no doubt? If it was, well played big brother! Mom even confirmed! I guess I have been under the wrong impression my entire life!" Having to confirm pallbearers, I called up Jonathan a little later. After he agreed to stand up for Jim, he asked me about the obituary.

"Well, I wanted to show Jim's personality in the obituary and when he said the son of Art and Corrie, I knew I had to. Sorry," I said waiting cautiously for his reply.

I didn't need to wait long as he laughed, "Well played Joanne. Well played." I let out the breath I was holding in as a smile spread across my lips.

That night, as I lay in bed by myself, I thought of the few times I slept without Jim during our marriage. It was only a handful of times. As tears trickled out of the corner of my eyes and down my cheeks it was not long before I fell into an exhausted, medicated sleep.

Think about it.

Who would be your pallbearers? Pick six people (and a few extra in case someone you ask, declines). Keep these names on file. In this file also keep an updated picture of yourself that can be given to the funeral home for all the announcements and bulletins. While you're at it, why not start putting together a picture file of your life? You can add pictures every year. This will save time for those whom you have left behind. (And you get to pick the best pictures.)

Visitation Surprise

FRIDAY MORNING, DESIREE, Elly, and Melissa went to Staples in Stratford to print the bulletins. They also brought more than ten photo albums of Jim's life to have on display at the church, and a few framed family photos from over the years. I sent along his cadet shirt and the jar of memories with extra pens and colourful recipe cards to put on the table for people to add their own memories, while they waited in line.

"Don't forget all those pies too!" I reminded them. Seeing that my Mom and Dad had also arrived at the house, I gave my Dad the job of picking up the KFC later that day, which I had ordered for supper between visitation times. I hoped I had ordered enough. Everyone else, after each quickly grabbing a sandwich, headed to the church for 1:00 pm.

At the church, we were greeted by the funeral home staff, Jeff, Angelena, and Curtis. As I hung up my coat, I admired how my girls had set up everything so neatly on the tables in the back foyer. Jeff then came to let me know what the plan was on their end, confirming what I was expecting.

"I forgot to ask you if I could get his ring back too?" I questioned.

"Now?" he said, a little worried.

"No, no, just at some point," I reassured him.

"Oh, sure, we can do that. Did you want to wear it tomorrow for the funeral?" he asked.

"No, that's fine. I can pick it up sometime next week."

With that figured out, he encouraged me to go to the front of the church, where Jim's body lay in the open casket. I walked slowly, feeling numb. I know some of my kids were with me, but I don't remember who. Together we stood there looking at the shell. "Lord, help us through this," I prayed silently as tears slid down my cheeks. These tears weren't for Jim, but for those of us who had to go on without him. Feeling no reason to stay long as I knew *he* wasn't there, I turned and headed to the back. Others took their turns in silence. Some others chose not to, which was okay too.

Later as the casket was closed at the front of the church, Pastor Martin prayed with the whole family. As people started to arrive shortly before 2:00 pm, the overhead projector started to display the photos the kids had collected beforehand. We arranged ourselves at the front, facing the closed casket, my older children on my right with their spouses and the younger ones on my left, with my parents on the end. In different pews sat my siblings and Jim's siblings along with their kids, greeting and talking to those who walked past. Again, I felt sad for Jim's parents as they couldn't make it, but I knew this would have been very hard for them too.

It was good to all be together here. It was good to see our friends from years gone by and those we see every week. Grown men told me they remembered Jim as their cadet counsellor. Others remembered him as their youth elder. I was meeting friends of my kids who I had heard about but never met in person. It surprised me to see so many people. I thought many would have stayed home because of the COVID restrictions.

It was good to tell different parts of our story. Desiree said, "It was a very special week for our family, it felt like we weren't alone. We were all in it together, sharing memories and keeping the mood light, following the tone that Dad had set. It felt warm and inviting and there was so much support from family and friends coming through the revolving door."

As things slowed down, we hurried downstairs for the KFC my dad had picked up. As I saw all the family sitting, I realized I hadn't ordered enough. I went over to my friend Jennifer and her daughter Emily, who had agreed to serve dinner and clean up, and told her my grave mistake.

Smiling, she said, "There is more than enough Joanne. Sit down and eat. You still have a long night ahead." I was confused but thankful. Silently thanking the Lord for however he used the "two fish" (or chicken) to feed my multitude.

After we ate, one of the kids came to tell me our friend and old neighbour Deb from Swansons Jewelry was here. I then remembered the call I had made to her yesterday, agreeing to meet here. She had brought with her a longer chain for me to display the "J" charm Jim gave me this past Christmas. It was just the right length to hang the charm as a necklace with my new dress.

After a short visit with her and her husband, I was again called back to join the receiving line as people were trickling back in for the 6:00–8:00 shift. Soon we were again engulfed in a sea of faces. There were those dearly loved people who were as crazy as we were and chose to homeschool their children. There were also those Jim had worked with in the past and neighbours from the different neighbourhoods we had lived in. The line kept coming and coming. Many memories were shared, we laughed, some of us shed tears. But they were happy tears. I kept looking over to my right to see who was coming down the line so I had time to mentally figure out who they were and how I might know them. I would try to catch bits of the conversations they were having with my kids, to help jog my memory. With some people, I just wanted to order tea and have a good visit. It was like watching your life walk by you in the faces of others.

In the midst of all this, someone tapped me on my left shoulder. Thinking it was one of my kids, I turned. I saw a man, and to his left, a step behind, was a woman. I knew these people but couldn't remember where from. Two seconds later it slammed into my brain. Jan and Wilma! I launched into Jan's arms and all my pent-up emotion came springing forward with sob after sob as we held each other. I pulled away and reached for Wilma, holding her close we too cried together. When I finally got control of myself, I asked what they were doing back here and how long they were staying.

"We couldn't sit at home and watch online. That wouldn't be right. We had to come back. We will talk more later; people are waiting for you. We are not going anywhere," Jan said as he gently encouraged me back to my position in line.

Apologizing to those who were waiting for me, I couldn't help but smile, "Our friends from Holland. They were just here two weeks ago. They came back!" Later I found out that Jan had contacted my brother James. James and his family had arrived with everyone else at 1:00 pm, but he left sometime during dinner to go to the airport. They travelled light, knowing it would just be for two nights, and figured they could get through the airport faster. Their flight was a little delayed. They didn't know if they would make it in time. Thankfully, the lineup for visitation went on for an additional two hours. They had plenty of time.

At the end of the night, the funeral home staff moved the casket to the back of the church, preparing to bring it back to the funeral home. As we were all preparing to leave, Jan asked about it, not knowing the custom in Canada. I asked him if he and Wilma would like to say goodbye to Jim. They did. I called Angelena and explained the situation. Happy to accommodate us, they set the coffin up by the back wall and reopened it. I encouraged them to say their goodbyes.

"You come with us? Yes?" Jan asked while taking hold of my left arm. With Wilma on my right, we walked up to the casket together. Following their lead, I waited. After a time, they looked at me and nodded. We slowly walked away and I thanked Angelena. Knowing they must be exhausted, we agreed to let them sleep in at the hotel they had booked in Stratford. My brother was lending them a car for the few days they were here so they would meet us back at the church in the morning at about 10:00. My feet ached as I walked back to the car in my high-calf black boots, heading home with some of the kids.

Funeral

I HAD TO smile while doing the chicken chores the next day, as I thought about seeing Jan and Wilma again later that morning. I still couldn't believe that they had come back. After the chickens were fed and watered and the eggs collected, I went back into the house to have my breakfast and prepare for the day.

By 10:00 am we were back at the church, gathering as a family down in the fellowship hall. Jeff was organizing us in groups as Jim's mom arrived. She drove herself after a friend came to stay with Dad. When it was time to go upstairs, I was again shocked to see how many people were there. But I was extremely thankful, to say the least. I know Jim had made an impact on many people, people I didn't even know. That was evident when I read over the comments left on the obituary site and the funeral registration book.

At 11:00 am I walked down the aisle with my two youngest boys, Calvin and Joshua, beside me. Following us were my two youngest daughters, Elly and Melissa. Then came Christina's family, Victoria and her boyfriend Seth, followed by Nathan, Nicolas, Desiree, and Derek, with their respective families. We were all guided to sit on the right, while Jim's mom and siblings with their family were guided across from us on the left. Behind them came my parents and siblings and their families. Jan and Wilma sat behind James.

Pastor Martin welcomed everyone, and we began by singing one of the songs Jim chose, "A Mighty Fortress is our God." Desiree, Elly, and Melissa went up to support each other as they took turns telling funny stories about their dad, each written by a different sibling. They ended with a thank you to everyone who supported us along this journey. Jim's oldest nephew, Joel, Julia's son, read messages written by Jim's three siblings. This ended with Jonathan publicly declaring that Mom confirmed Jim was the favourite son, to which everyone chuckled.

Jessica, Nathan's wife, came up and shared her beautiful voice, singing Jim's request, "I Love to Tell the Story."

Pastor Martin read Psalm 127 and 2 Timothy 4: 6–8, *"For I am already being poured out like a drink offering, and the time has come for my departure. I have fought the good fight, I have finished the race, I have kept the faith. Now there is in store for me the crown of righteousness, which the Lord, the righteous Judge, will award to me on that day—and not only to me, but also to all who have longed for his appearing."* After this reading we sang, "Rock of Ages."

Pastor Martin went on to encourage us to continue telling our stories of Jim as that is how we will honour his life. Having lost Jim, these stories are a way to keep him alive in our hearts. I agreed with Pastor Martin. It meant so much to us when people would tell us stories of Jim.

"We know where Jim has gone," said Pastor Martin. "He told us and we saw it in the life he lived. He lived his Christian life in his everyday life, finding joy at work and in all the other activities he did. Jim was not defined by the work he did, as he loved his family and made time to serve in the church." Taking the bible passage that Jim kept at the table beside his chair (2 Corinthians 4:16–18), Pastor Martin explained it for those who maybe didn't understand.

> *"Therefore we do not lose heart. Though outwardly we are wasting away, yet inwardly we are being renewed day by day. For our light and momentary troubles are achieving for us an eternal glory that far outweighs them all. So we fix our eyes not on what is seen, but on what is unseen. For what is seen is temporary, but what is unseen is eternal."*

"What is seen in this life is our hands, our feet, family and friends, each day. What is unseen is our soul and what God is doing in heaven. The chariots of God come down to take his people home. Focus on what is unseen. That is having faith," he taught. "Faith is like a furnace... it turns on when it is cold inside.... When life is going well, we might not focus on faith. When life gets hard, it's faith that kicks in and warms us."

We must remember that the challenges of today are momentary. They are just for a little while. After death is eternity. Where will you spend eternity?

For the last song, I chose, "My Friends May You Grow in Grace." I remember that years ago Desiree's girls' small bible study group sang this song to each other after every meeting. Jim and I loved the words. I wanted to send all our friends away from this place with that same blessing of learning more about Jesus each and every day.

As the service came to a close, Jeff came to the front and respectfully led the coffin out with the help of his son. He instructed me to follow behind him. I stepped into the aisle and waited for Jim's mom. Together we walked to the back as the family followed us out. Once at the back the five boys and Jonathan walked beside the casket and helped lift it into the waiting car. Once they drove away, we all quietly and somberly re-entered the church, our eyes glistening in tears. Mom was in a hurry to leave; she didn't want to talk to anyone. It took Jonathan and me a few minutes to help her locate her coat. During this time, it was decided that Jonathan and Joe (Mary's husband) would get mom home safely and come right back. Meanwhile, the others had made their way downstairs for the luncheon. When I arrived, everyone was standing back against the walls and the tables were piled high with food. Why was no one eating? I thought to myself.

Angelena from the funeral home, gracefully approached me and whispered, "We are ready to begin."

Leaning in so she could hear my whispered tone, I asked, "Begin what?"

She smiled warmly at me. "The luncheon," she said, stepping back so I could pass. It then dawned on me as I realized what was going on. Feeling sorry that I had kept everyone waiting, I headed to the table. I wondered if my perpetually hungry boys had snuck a bun or square without someone noticing.

Thankfully, I got to go first and was able to almost get one bun down before people came to talk to me, putting an end to my lunch. But that was okay as I got to see more people that I didn't see the day before. Cousins of mine and cousins of Jim's, all of which I have not seen in years, came to give their condolences. It was so good to see everyone. I noticed my kids sitting at tables or standing, each with their own group of friends or with their spouse's families, all who came out to support them. It was a beautiful world full of activity that I wish could have lasted longer. I greatly enjoyed the stories of Jim, and hoped some of them were being written on the cards that the girls left on the tables around the room to add to "Papa's Jar of Memories." Happy memories, good memories. This was a time to thank God for the years that we had to enjoy him.

As the last people trickled out of the church, we were trying to divide up the many flower arrangements that had arrived. I invited the whole family to hang out at our house. Jim's family thanked me but thought they better go hang out with Mom and Dad. I understood and made sure they took a flower arrangement for mom. Meanwhile, the rest of the family headed to my house, along with Jan and Wilma. Just like the week before, the house was booming with activity. Grandkids ran the halls and played with toys or puzzles that were dumped out across the floor. Some of my kids started a game on the dining room table while others sat on the couches.

I noticed Jan and Wilma sitting quietly beside me watching the flurry of activity. Jan finally leaned over and said for only me to hear, "This is not the family we met a few weeks ago."

"No, but *this* is the family Jim wanted to show you," I said, with a huge smile, sweeping my arms open. While gesturing to the full room, one of the grandkids went squealing past us, with an uncle in hot pursuit. Jan smiled with me.

Eventually everyone made their way back to their own homes later in the afternoon for a good sleep before a quiet Sunday. Everyone knew that before long Monday would be upon them and it would be time return to work and school. My brother and I made arrangements to return Jan and Wilma to the Toronto airport. He asked if I would like to come along. I thanked them, looking forward to visiting as much as possible with Jan and Wilma. Later that night Jan and Wilma headed back to their hotel room with a promise to return in the morning to do church online.

By the next morning, however, we had changed our minds and decided to watch the funeral service once again. This time we could talk about any questions they had about our services being different than theirs. They were astonished to find out that Jim had not been buried yesterday.

"This is Canada," I laughed. "The ground is frozen. The bigger cemeteries have a machine that heats the ground so it is easier to dig a hole, but this is a small cemetery. We have to wait until after April to bury him. There is a place north of here where the body goes to cold storage until then."

"So do you have another service then?" they asked.

"Yes, a small one at the cemetery. But our minister will be on sabbatical—like a holiday. So I will be asking a good friend of Jim's who also preaches in our church sometimes. Are you going to come back then too?" I laughed.

"No, I think it will be a few years before we come again. But you can come to Holland!"

Hearing this, Elly—my world traveller—piped up, "Yeah mom! We can go together!"

"I don't know if I'm ready for that just yet," I answered. "I will come, but I will wait a little bit first." Looking over at Elly, I could see the gears turning as she smiled, already planning our trip

After lunch, I joined Wilma in the back seat so we could get in some good visiting in the short time we had left. We laughed, joked, and even shed a few tears on that drive—all the things that make a good friendship. Ours is one of those rare friendships where you can just pick up where you left off, as if there had been no days in between.

We found James and his wife Jane in Hamilton where we had agreed to meet, before carrying on to the Toronto airport. Upon arriving at the airport, we were only able to drop them off at the door because of the new COVID rules. We hugged each other quickly, and thanked each other. We then left them at the airport and James pulled the van back into traffic, heading toward Fullarton. Before I knew it, we arrived at home, having had a great conversation. Needing a break from driving, they stayed for a short visit before taking the two-hour drive home.

After waving goodbye from the driveway, I re-entered the house with a sigh. It was one of those of those energy and stress-relieving sighs. Walking through the house, this house that had so many people coming and going over the past week and more, I breathed in the smell of all the flower arrangements that were left here and there. The organizer in me felt a need to get my house back in order, but that would have to wait until tomorrow. Tonight, I needed to talk to the kids who were left behind, the ones I was still the primary caregiver for. I needed to see how they were doing.

Paperwork

MONDAY, I CALLED my life insurance broker, Roger, to let him know that Jim had passed. We talked for a bit before he told me he would email me the forms to fill out and asked that I also send a copy of the will and the death certificate. This was yet another form that needed to go to Dr. Thornton for her to confirm cancer as his cause of death. Later that day I went and brought more paperwork to the doctor's office. While there, I picked up the long-term disability paperwork, and wondered if we still needed it. I was gaining new respect for doctors, considering all the paperwork they have to fill out.

At one point I noticed Jim's book, *A Father's Legacy*, on the table beside his chair. Taking a seat in his chair, I laid the book on my lap and let it fall open about two-thirds of the way in to where his pen marked his last entry. On page 126 the question asked, "What are the things you hope your children have learned from you?" Underneath he had started writing, "The most important is love and trust our Lord and Saviour. Just to go with that, to worship Him in truth and… " He hadn't finished. There was ink on the page as if he had fallen asleep with the pen hovering above the page. But having read the words I knew what he was trying to say, so I finished it for him.

"Dad (Papa) fell asleep writing this, never getting to finish, but I, Mom (Grandma) remembered this from his loved Promise Keepers cassette tape… John 4:23–24, "*Yet a time is coming and has now come when the true worshipers will worship the Father in spirit and truth, for they are the kind of worshipers the Father seeks. God is spirit, and his worshippers must worship in spirit and in truth.*"

Victoria visited a few nights later. We ended up talking about the quilt we were going to make out of dad's funny t-shirts and other clothes. As we went through the clothes I separated them into piles, one for the quilt and one for those that I would wear, such as some of his good sweatshirts. I gave the girls back the university sweatshirt and t-shirts they had got him as Christmas gifts, for them to wear to remember their dad. I would ask if anyone from work wanted his many, many Premier shirts. Or maybe the girls would want to make one into a pillow. Throwing his underwear out and giving the boys some of his belts, I had finally emptied everything out. People said that would be hard, but for me it was fun doing it with my daughter. We laughed at the stories, especially when I told her about the time he packed for himself for an overnight stay at my parents. The next morning he was wearing his plaid shorts and a plaid button-up shirt. The girls and I just stood there staring.

"That's all you took?'" we asked.

"Yeah, what's wrong with it? I think it looks good. It even matches. Plaid and plaid," he said so proudly.

"No dad. This is bad!" the girls said, trying not to laugh and shaking their heads in disappointment. "How can we take you out in public?" They were not looking forward to walking around Niagara Falls with their friend from Germany with their dad dressed like he was. So, once we got to the Falls, the girls and I found the cheapest t-shirt shop and bought him a solid grey Niagara Falls t-shirt. When we met him and the boys down by the park we made a b-line to him and forced him to wear the new shirt.

"But I like this one," he stressed, rubbing his belly and trying to hide his smile. The girls tried to wrestle it off of him. "Leave my nice shirt alone or I'll call the police on you. Police! Police! These girls are stealing my shirt," he said, now full-out laughing with the rest of us. Trying to change our tactic, I pulled out the new shirt and started pointing out all the good things about the new one.

"Look, it matches better. You can look like the tourist that you are. See, it has the words Niagara Falls on it." Seeing this was not working, I put my hands on my hips and ordered him to take off the shirt. To which he cowered, with a smirk on his face and took off the plaid button-up shirt, changing it for this new t-shirt.

Victoria and I laughed at the story, making sure we had the plaid shirt with the plaid shorts and the solid Niagara Falls shirt. We made a few other sets to go with certain memories. Then there were the t-shirts that had different sayings on them, which he had received as gifts from different kids. We discussed how we would attach his Sunday tie to his light blue shirt.

"Where is the bright blue shirt he wore for the weddings?" she asked.

"He is wearing it," I said matter-of-factly.

"What do you mean he is wearing it?" she asked, confused.

"We buried him in it," I said as the meaning sunk in.

"Oh," she said as I burst out laughing, and she joined in. It seemed easier to go through his clothes as I knew these pieces were going in the quilt. They were still here in the house if I wanted them. They just were not in the closet.

Then I went out, making my first purchase for our home without Jim's approval. I bought a curtain for my closet which had never had doors before. Now I couldn't see how empty it was.

Think about it

Cleaning out closets can be a hard step in the grieving process. It is easier to do with someone with you, someone who will listen to your stories.

If you are helping someone clean out a loved one's closet, you need to sit back and let them work through it. Listen to their stories, let them cry. Do not do it for them, as this is a huge part of the grieving process. Don't rush them. Wait until they are ready.

The following Wednesday I had an appointment with Jeff Lockhart to go through some paperwork. He had instructed me to bring along Jim's passport, his health card, our marriage certificate, my social insurance number, and a void cheque. Having this list of things written in the little brown notebook, I tucked it, along with the items, into my purse. When I arrived at the funeral home, I rang the doorbell, feeling confident that I could do this on my own.

Once again, I found myself sitting across the desk from Jeff. With a smile, he handed me a bag with Jim's t-shirt, followed by a small navy-blue velvet bag. He informed me that it held Jim's ring. I accepted it but didn't open it. I didn't trust my heart at that moment. He then held out an open flat shoebox-style box. Inside lay a dark book with Jim's obituary photo on the front behind protective clear plastic.

"That is the register book with all the signatures from those who came to the visitation and the funeral. In the back are pages with the messages that were sent on the website and a list of those who ordered flowers." He went on to explain how to send electronic thank you cards and gave suggestions for the wording. He said I should try to have them done by next week. With the simplicity of electronic thank you cards, it seemed very doable.

"Did you get any more cards?" I asked. "We seem to be missing a few."

"Yes, they are in that box, under the book," he said pointing to the box in my lap. I looked down and noticed them peeking out underneath the book. I thanked him. I made notes in the brown book as we set the date of the interment for May 14 at 1:30 pm. I offered to contact John and Mary to let them know about the date for the grave opening.

We then went on to the government paperwork. We worked through the forms to cancel Jim's passport, his health card, and his driver's license. We also filled out the form for a Death Benefit with Service Canada which is a one-time payout. I was so happy when we just motored on through this paperwork. Jeff knew which boxes to fill, and a lot of the information was the same for each form. In no time we were finished and I headed off to the post office to get a tracking number for the passport. Then I was off to Service Ontario to drop off the health card and cancel the driver's license. Later at home, I wrote the boys' social insurance numbers in the highlighted sections of the Death Benefit form. After closing up the envelope, I brought it straight to the mailbox across the street. Done! Well, almost. I still had to deal with all the regular bills (sigh).

Later at home, I pulled Jim's ring out of the little bag and put it on my middle finger on my left hand, looking down at it with dry eyes. Then I turned to the registry book. As I went down the list, I read the names of people I didn't remember seeing there. Then there were other names that I couldn't read as they had written their signature as if it was a legal document. From now on, I will neatly print my name in these books when I go to a funeral. A signature defeats the purpose.

More Paperwork

THE NEXT AFTERNOON, I was off to see the lawyer. This was a meeting I wasn't comfortable doing by myself. Messaging the two boys who were to be the executors of our estate, I apologized for the short notice and asked if they could join me. Surprisingly, they both were able to make it work. I kept hearing Jim in my head saying, "You don't need me. You are capable of doing this on your own." I hated it when he did that in the past. I wanted to have his help. But I guess it was one of those things that helped me be a stronger person.

Later that afternoon, in Ben's office, together with two knowledgeable sons, we went through the will.

"So, Joanne, you get everything," Ben said. Now that was simple. "But there are a few things we should talk about as you go through the process of figuring things out. First, I tell all my clients, do *not* open an estate account with the bank. It is not in your best interest at all." I wrote that in big letters in my brown notebook. *No estate account.*

He asked if we had life insurance on the mortgage. I knew right off that we didn't, as we had just renewed in January, and Jim would have never been able to get it at that point. He suggested I find out my current mortgage rate and what the rate was on a GIC. If it was a better GIC rate than my mortgage, he encouraged me to invest the money instead of paying off the mortgage right away. That way I could make some money from it.

I told him that I had called the Life Insurance broker and we had that ball rolling. Ben then said that whenever I was ready, he could change the house into my name. To do that he would need a death certificate. I reached down to the bag I had beside me, the one carrying all the legal papers I thought I might need, including the death certificates. I handed him one. He took it and set it to the side, folding his hands on our folder in front of him.

213

"Do you have any questions?"

"Yes, what do I do about cancelling our business?"

"Is it active?"

"No. Well, two, three years ago, we did one weekend milking but nothing since."

"Okay, so you need to see your accountant."

"I don't have one because Jim did all our own income tax filing online. We thought that was easier. Can you suggest anyone?" I asked. The boys had been quiet for the most part, just listening and taking things in. One now piped up and suggested his accountant.

"She is really good and easy to work with," he said.

"Actually, I was going to suggest her also, as I use her myself. Just wait till next week, though, because I have to get my stuff to her first," Ben said, laughing.

"Well, I think I'm good for this last income tax year, as Jim and I did it together two weeks ago," I informed him.

"I would suggest that you get an accountant for a couple of years, at least until you get all the details figured out. There will be extra things to figure out for this coming year. Trust me, it will be worth your while," he encouraged. I wrote down the accountant's name and number.

"What about identity theft? Jim has a Twitter account, and I don't have his password for that."

"You can go on the internet and google how to close an account for someone who has died. It should say how to do it. I haven't done it before," he explained. The boys agreed that I should be able to do it online.

"Joanne, if you get any flak from anyone when you call, just hang up and call back. The next person will probably not give you a hard time. There just seems to be one in every crowd. But if they are still giving you a hard time, just let me know. We can put something on our letterhead, and they usually comply right away." He said this with a smile. "Any other questions?" he asked. I shook my head, looking left and right at the boys. They also didn't have any questions. "If you think of anything else, please feel free to contact me at any time." With that information, the boys and I thanked Ben for his time and left the building. On the street, I thanked them for coming with me.

"No problem, Mom."

"I just didn't want to miss any important information. I also thought it best if you two know what is going on since you're in charge of the estate."

"No, all is good, Mom," they responded. After a quick hug from both we headed in our separate directions.

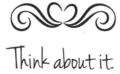

Think about it

It is important to have a good accountant, someone you trust. There is special paperwork to do for your loved one's final income tax return, and the accountant will know all the ins and outs. If you have a business to close, they know how to deal with this also. It will be one less thing you need to think about while you are grieving.

A week later, I made a decision. I needed to have a day designated for going through all of Jim's paperwork. At the time, I was finding myself on a call or texting with a minimum of three children a day. And you know how long moms and daughters can talk on the phone. It wasn't always the same children, they were gracious enough to rotate. But something needed to be done! I sent out a message on the FamJam, "I love you all dearly, but tomorrow I will not be answering any phone calls or messages. I need to get some paperwork done around here." Once I finished teaching Joshua the next morning, I went up to my desk with my laptop, my cell phone, and the brown notebook.

Opening the filing drawer, I took a deep breath as my hand ran past the *auto* file. I knew we already moved everything into my name, so I moved on. But then my eye caught the word "motorcycle." Oh no, we forgot to change the ownership of the motorcycle. I would have to talk to Ben about that. I made a note in the brown notebook, and then continued.

Doctor. I called the eye doctor and the dentist to let them know Jim had passed. Our other doctors already knew. The dentist said they had already taken care of it, as they check the obituaries.

Heat. I called the place where we got our furnace oil and explained that Jim passed. I wanted to know what I had to do to remove Jim's name from the account. I was told to go online and follow the prompts to fill out a form to have it changed. With the laptop in front of me, I made sure I did it while I was on the phone with them.

Water heater rental. I called them and they were able to remove Jim's name from the account themselves. Easy-peasy.

Insurance. They would need a copy of the death certificate and the will. I remembered that Ben had suggested I not give out a copy of the whole will, just the front page. I went down to the printer and scanned both forms to have on my laptop if anyone else needed a copy.

Mortgage. I compared our current interest rate with the Bank's GIC rate online. It would be better for me to keep my mortgage and invest the money. I moved on.

Phone. I called and they had no problem taking Jim's name off our landline. However, I couldn't get through to his cellular provider, so I set that one aside. (I was able to do it a few days later by phone.)

Educational Savings Plans. I explained the situation *again* and received condolences. "I'm so sorry, ma'am." Again. The lady asked if I had a life insurance policy with the kids' scholarships.

"Pardon?" I asked. She repeated herself. I didn't know the answer. She looked it up. Apparently, the remainder of the kids' scholarships will be paid up as we had insurance. That was a pleasant surprise. But of course, I had to fill out some forms for that too, again sending along a copy of the will and a death certificate. Thankfully she walked me through all that also.

Visa. I wanted to do this one in person, as it was his credit card. I was given a second card to use under his name. It doesn't expire for a few years, so maybe I can still use it. It has always been paid up.

Email. I didn't have any magazine subscriptions to cancel, but there were some emails that we were getting on our shared account that I wanted to cancel. While I cancelled these, I went through some of the other junk email. For most of the emails, I could just scroll to the bottom of the email and click "unsubscribe." But some were not that easy.

Rifling through his wallet to see if there was anything else I needed to cancel, I found his library card. So, I made that phone call. The other cards were nothing to cancel but held some memories. Moving his Tim Hortons card to my wallet, I couldn't help but smile. I was remembering our Tim Hortons date nights in St. Marys. They were always cut short when the local retired farmers would come to join Jim at the table. He would just shrug and smile at me, and I knew that our date night was over. That's when we started to go to McDonald's in Exeter; no one knew him there. Then there was the nearly empty gift card his mom gave us for a dinner out at Swiss Chalet. As I looked through all the pockets, I found his taped-together SIN card, his driver's license, and his hospital card. In a back pocket, I pulled out a very worn, small rectangular paper. I remembered this paper. One New Year's party a number of years ago, at our neighbour Nick and Kirsten's, they had everyone write down their favourite bible verse and what it meant to them. They then had everyone put their papers into a bowl, and they mixed them up. This is the one Jim picked out that a young lady named Alexia had written. As Jim read it aloud, we all laughed as it seemed appropriate for him, but he had taken it to heart and kept it:

Enlarge the place of your tent; Stretch out the curtains of your dwellings, spare not; lengthen your pegs. For you will spread abroad to the right and to the left and your descendants will possess nations and will resettle the desolate cities (Isaiah 54:2–3). In her own words she explained, "This means that God is about to give you a promise to expand your faith, etc. because this promise is coming!"

Jim's Stuff

NOW FOR THOSE chickens. After gathering everything I needed, I began shovelling out the condo. The more I shovelled, the more my asthma kicked in. Before I knew it, my heart was pounding, and my chest was tight. Forcing myself to finish the small coop, I was soon sitting out on a chair, in the fresh air catching my breath. As I did so, I texted Nathan, "I think it's time you got your chickens."

Soon came the reply, "Why, what happened?"

"My asthma. I was trying to clean out the condo."

"Well, I have to make a coop yet."

"That's fine. Take your time. The condo is clean now."

"LOL, okay, Mom."

Think about it

Your loved one's interests may not be, and most likely are not, your interests. You do not need to keep doing their hobbies. Give yourself permission to let them go. Yes, it can be very hard, wanting to keep their passions/hobbies alive, but it becomes one more thing on your plate that you didn't have before. You have permission to let it go.

Every day the mailbox had at least one or two new cards. Some were just signed. Others had assurances of prayer. The ones that meant the most included a story about Jim. Those were treasures. A friend who had lost her husband about ten years before shared Isaiah 54:5, a verse she clung to. *"For your Maker is your husband—the LORD Almighty is his name—the Holy One of Israel is your Redeemer; he is called the God of all the earth."*

Who wouldn't want a close relationship with the creator of all the earth? I decided then and there that this would be my verse also. As I lay awake at night thinking of this concept, I realized that I should have been thinking this way for years. I should have been turning to God with my stress in life first, not Jim. I guess we all need to get to a point when we realize it's important to love and cherish our spouses, and our best friends, but our dependency should be on God alone. He will never let us down. As I lay there looking at the wall or ceiling, I would thank the Lord for the time I was able to have with Jim. The good times, and yes, the rough times too, as they are what made us grow into the people we became. As someone wrote in another card, "God still has a purpose for you here, Joanne." Now as I try to look ahead, I talk (pray) to my new husband.

"Lord, what do you need me to do here for you? Why have you left me behind? To write a book? To help someone deal with their stuff so they can find you? Lord, show me where I need to be. Open my eyes; help me feel it in my heart. Give me the joy and peace that can only be found in doing your work."

While talking to the friend who gave me my new verse, she suggested I try signing up for GriefShare. She had found it helpful in the past. It is a grief support group where you meet with others while working through your grief. She mentioned that, since COVID, they have a new program that you can sign up for to receive a devotional a day for a year. I decided to try it, since there were no support groups in my area running at the time. In one of the first emails I received, I read that everyone's journey is very different, and we are not to compare ourselves to others. I was noticing that myself, even within my own family.

I felt like I was hovering on a fine line, dealing with the past while looking to the future. I was asking questions like, "Who am I?" or "What do I do now?" I had dreams of the future which included Jim. That part was now gone, and I was feeling like my future was gone with him. Jim and I were planning motorcycle trips. Now my driver is gone, and so is that dream. Now I have to make new dreams. I don't feel like it today, but slowly, with God's help, I know I can move in that direction. I am learning who I am now without that *huge* part of me.

The day came when I bit the bullet and entered the bank that held our visa card. It hadn't worked on the past two transactions, so I wondered if word leaked out. The friendly clerk behind the counter looked up the card online and didn't know why it wasn't working. She called over another person, and he also didn't see why it wouldn't be working. I was then brought to another employee who deals with credit cards. As I sat in that office, the walls seemed to close in and I was overwhelmed by a need to get out of there. How could I get out? My mind raced. The lady behind the desk, I'm sure, was friendly, but everything on me was bristling. I had never felt this way before. I was angry at her, and she had done nothing wrong.

"Well, Mrs. Schreuders, I see this is your husband's card. Legally, I am not able to talk to you about it. Maybe we could set up an appointment for him?" she politely asked. Well, from somewhere deep down inside, my alter ego came rising to the surface.

"Well, good luck with that. He is dead," I said rudely. Shocked that that came out of my mouth, yet amazed that I didn't feel regret, I clamped it shut while still fighting the feeling of wanting to run. As her head flew up to look at me, I could hear the angel and devil arguing, each on a shoulder, their voices bouncing through my head. She took a minute to process my sharp words.

"I'm sorry for your loss Mrs. Schreuders."

"Listen, I just need a credit card, and I need to find the best rate. The card my husband had is the best rate we have seen in years. Can you give me one with this rate?"

"No, this is a very unique card. Let me see what we might have for you," she said, turning back to her computer to slowly search her screen, clicking here and there. Finally, she found a couple of options and started to explain them in great detail. I know she was just trying to do her job, but I needed to get out of there. However, I forced myself to sit politely.

"Okay, thank you for your time. I will take that information with me as I do some more research."

"Ma'am, I think you might be best off just going to your own bank and getting a credit card there. They know your bank account figures and we don't. Later, once you have built up credit, then you can search again." I agreed with her and took one last moment to thank her very much for her time before turning and fleeing the building. Once outside, I just wanted to run and run and run. Instead, I forced myself to walk slowly and let the tears fall where they may. I felt utterly defeated. Making my way to my bank on the other side of the street, I regained composure before entering, wondering if now was really a good time. Having cleaned my face with my shirt sleeve, I hoped for the best and entered through the door. A few minutes later, I was directed to the lady who helps you apply for credit cards. After only a few minutes of data entry, she was able to tell me that my new credit card would be in the mail shortly. I thanked her and left in a civil manner, very proud of the way I handled myself the second time around.

A few days later, still mulling over my surprising behaviour at the bank, I opened that day's GriefShare devotional email. I learned that grief can come out in unexplained moments of anger. They had suggestions on how to deal with it. I was eager to read on. I hoped to never have that experience again.

As the days passed, many people messaged asking if they could come for a visit. I would welcome them but asked if they would be up to walking with me. They would walk with me not only physically but also emotionally, as I would tell them many times the story of what we went through. After some time had passed, I realized I hadn't inquired how they or their families were. I came to realize that these were true friends. I loved each of them for being there for me. When I needed to talk, they had graciously listened.

Think about it

As you watch those around you grieve, it hurts, and you want them to be better. You might want to fix it. But they each have to go through the process on their own. *Nothing* you do can make it go faster or make it go away. So please don't give up on them. The best thing you can do for them is to quietly listen to them as they process aloud. *"Carry each other's burdens, and in this way you will fulfill the law of Christ"* (Galatians 6:2).

One day I wanted to send an encouragement card to a few people in the church who were on our daily prayer list. I grabbed a few cards out of the drawer and set them on the table to look over. I wanted to find the right words for the right person. After opening a few, thinking about which would be the best, I reached for another one. And there at the bottom of the card, slamming into my heart, was Jim's signature. The sobs came suddenly and violently. I had always given Jim a small stack of cards to read through to help me pick the perfect one before we would sign and mail it off. He most likely signed one of the extra ones. But I knew without a shadow of a doubt, that God had him sign it. God needed to tell me something. I wanted to know what it was, but my eyes were busy swimming. Laying the card down on the table, almost reverently, I allowed myself to cry till the tears were spent. When I could finally see again, I picked up the card, bracing myself. I read the words multiple times, trying to understand what God was trying to tell me.

> God will always give us the answers we need to live the life we are
> meant to live.
> All we need to do is search our hearts for the answers.
>
> (Signed) Jim

I then set it up on the shelf beside my bed for regular encouragement and something to ponder.

I decided to make a trip out to Living Waters Book & Toy store in Elmira. I wanted to find a new devotional book that the boys and I could do together. But I also hoped they might find some books that interested them. Elly asked to come along as she also had a short list of things she was looking for. So, off the four of us went; two very reluctantly. Upon arriving in this big store, I leisurely walked along the outside wall looking at pictures that might go well in my room. Then it happened. My eyes turned to a big picture mounted high on the wall of a path leading down to the beach. Jim's favourite spot. It had Psalm 16:11 written on it. I couldn't tear my eyes off it as the view started to swim in front of me. I finally moved on to find the grief section on the other side of the store. Here, I found a book by Phil Callaway called, *Laugh Like a Kid Again.* I remembered when Jim and I saw him in person. We really enjoying his work, so I decided to get the book. Seeing the Bible study section close by, I asked the boys, who were exasperated with me, to help find something. Calvin just stood there ready to complain, but Joshua, my thinker, knew that we could leave if he picked one. After a swift look over the rack, he picked up one and handed it to me.

"This one," he said with a big smile. Looking down into my hand I too smiled seeing the title, "Joshua." Knowing that any bible study would be fine, we took our books to the checkout. As it turned out, Joshua's pick was a very appropriate study for the time we were in. Joshua—the Bible Joshua—had to trust God when things didn't seem possible. He had to trust God completely, as we had to do now.

Soon I was back at Jeff Lockhart's office to pay for Jim's funeral with the life insurance money I had received. I also wanted to pay for my funeral, so my kids wouldn't have to worry about it. He had explained that the money would be put into an annuity in my name, reassuring me that it was a safe investment. Again, Jeff went over the details we had previously discussed. As I confirmed everything, only making slight changes that would make it easier for my kids, he tallied up the cost of my funeral. After he filled out the detailed contract, having me sign at the appropriate places, I gave him a void cheque for Funeral Plans Canada to take the total from my account. Before I left, Jeff let me know that the agreement and certificate for the annuity would be coming in the mail.

Think about it

Did you know that if you decide to pay for your funeral in advance, the money is put into an annuity in *your* name? In other words, the money is in a safe investment, not affected in any way if the funeral home would ever close. The interest you make on this money off-sets the increase in funeral costs. However, if the investment has not made enough interest, you should know that the funeral home covers the difference on the guaranteed portion. Although, chang-es made from the original pre-contract and disbursements, that aren't on the pre-contract, are not covered by the funeral home. Another interesting fact is that if the investment company folds, the Canadian Deposit Insurance Cooperation (CDIC) guarantees each of these investments. On the other hand, if the interest is good, making you more money than the cost of the funeral, the extra funds get put back into your estate or dispersed to the beneficiary.

A few days later I entered the accountant's office alone. I had with me a cloth bag of all my legal paperwork which she had asked for over the phone. When she joined me in the board room, we talked about Jim's business that we needed to close and what that would look like. She had me sign a few papers and accepted a copy of the death certificate as well as the first page of the will. We then discussed the disability tax credit and income tax forms. She would begin work on Jim's 2022 form for this year, only needing to do it until his March death date. I had a few more questions that she answered before I left it all in her capable hands.

The day before the interment, Rene (our best man) arrived at Toronto airport. Driving a rented car, he made his way to a Stratford hotel to drop off his stuff before heading to our house. Desiree and her family were staying at the house for the week-end to be close to tomorrow's activities. As we visited together, we also talked about Jim's motorcycle. I had sold it online to a nice man about Jim's age who just wanted a bike to tour around on. It seemed like a good fit. He was coming to pick it up in the morning, the only day he could get a trailer. Rene offered to be there when the guy came to pick it up.

"I think I will be okay. I was going to push it out in the driveway before he came. When he arrives, I'll give him the key and then I plan to go for a walk down by the river alone." I knew I would probably need a good cry. After catching up, Rene headed back to the hotel, and we to our beds with the promise of meeting at the house again at 10:00 in the morning. But before I headed to bed, I quietly snuck into the garage. By the light of the moon and a little nightlight in the ceiling outlet, I slowly approached the motorbike. My eyes started to mist. My hand slowly reached out to caress the leather seat where Jim would go to think. This was his happy place. Grabbing the handlebar, I swung my right leg over the seat and moved back to my seat. Not feeling safe perched up there on a parked bike, I slid back down to Jim's seat and the tears came faster. I closed my eyes and tried to imagine riding with him, holding him tight and watching him in the mirror with that huge smile on his face. Remembering the times we rode in the wind… and the rain. I smiled through tears as I remembered the windchimes.

"Lord, we were supposed to travel on this motorcycle, enjoying your creation," I whispered. I had a feeling watching the motorcycle leave tomorrow morning was going to be harder than burying him in the afternoon. Sobs shook my body. I sat there for a long time, even after my tears were spent. Finally, after climbing off slowly, I headed back to my bed. I realized that the tears were not spent just yet.

Interment

IT HAD BEEN eight and a half weeks without Jim and now the house was bustling with activity again. I went out to the garage to move the lonely bike, but instead I found a daughter, as I had been the night before. Mumbling an apology, I slipped back into the house, giving her the space she needed. A while later, seeing she was in the house again, I returned to the garage and opened the big garage door. Making my way back to the motorcycle with a specific goal in mind, I climbed on, grabbing both handles firmly. Slowly, I strained to push it out the door on my own power, finally propping it on its kickstand in the driveway. As I climbed back off the bike, I pocketed the key and went to close the garage door.

Later, while in the house, I noticed a truck and trailer pull into the driveway. With butterflies in my stomach, I put on my runners and headed out the door. Saying nothing, as he already knew what my day held, I handed the gentleman the key. He mouthed a thank you as I smiled a smile that didn't make it anywhere near my eyes. Not stopping, I turned and headed behind the house and to the path that led to the river. Here I walked, talking to God, asking for strength not only for myself, but for my family too, for whatever the day would hold.

When I returned to the house everyone was bustling about getting ready for the family photos that Rio, Jim's sister-in-law, was going to take. When she arrived, I showed her my "Wall of Fam," explaining how I wanted to display the photos she would take. With that in mind, we all trudged out to the small pine forest on the way to the river. Here we found a great place to take pictures while the kids ran around collecting dandelions. Instructing the kids to put down the flowers, we arranged them in family groups for the large family photo. Later we had to laugh, as there, just centre right at our feet, is a beautiful bouquet of bright yellow dandelions. It reminded us of Jim's passion to kill those weeds every spring with fierce intensity. This makes me laugh and love the photo even more.

With family everywhere once again, we had a self-serve lunch buffet. People took their plates to the living room, dining room, and even outside on the porch. With perfect timing, we headed to the cemetery to meet Jeff and Curtis Lockhart. Here, they gave me a short overview of what would be happening, and asked if I had any questions.

"No, but I have to let you know that two of the pallbearers have changed," I informed him. The youngest two boys had dug in their heels, this time would be too hard for them to do it. Having already done it once, I felt they could make that decision. I had asked Rene and our neighbour Nick to be the two substitutes. They were honoured to do it, but also willing to back out if the boys changed their minds.

"That's fine. I would have those of you acting as pallbearers to come to the back of the funeral coach and we'll proceed," he said smiling with ease. Looking around, we still needed to wait for some people.

Once everyone was there, we started, the older three boys, Jim's brother, and two friends representing the past and present. They walked in unison bringing the casket to its place over the grave. Jim's friend Stan officiating, began, only to stop shortly after starting, as another car drove up.

Once everyone was settled again, Stan continued, talking about being Jim's youth elder all those years ago. He also talked about some of his more recent visits and how the family was so important to Jim. Jim wanted them all to find Jesus as their own personal Saviour. As I stood there, I could hear the sniffles and sobs of my children behind me. I closed my eyes as a tear rolled down, another soon to follow. I looked out to the fields beyond, trying to picture Jim working all those fields around this cemetery when we had our own business years ago. This was the right choice for the cemetery. He was right. I smiled. Trying to bring my thoughts back to the present, I wiped away my tears. Stan, having concluded, brought us together in prayer. Once he finished, we all moved to the side as a gentleman came forward to lower the casket. I found myself beside Jennifer, as we had all shifted.

"I feel we should sing," she said quietly. I knew she was right.

"What song?" I asked.

"Did he have a favourite?" she asked, both of us still watching the casket being prepared. I was silent for a moment flailing through song titles in my head. Stopping short at the most obvious one, one we wouldn't need music for.

"'Living for Jesus', the cadet theme song!" we looked at each other then and smiled. Suddenly excited, probably because I had something to do, I went to where my kids stood and told them what we were going to do. I positioned myself back beside the person I felt could hold a tune better than me, and Jennifer started us off as they started to lower the coffin. At first, it was just Jennifer and I singing, but slowly others joined us.

Once the casket was in place we slowly turned and walked away, hugging and encouraging each other on the way.

Getting into Jim's truck, I slid behind the wheel, with Rene in the passenger seat and three kids in the backseat. I waited as a tractor came down the road toward us. As it came closer, I noticed it was one of the farmers that Jim had worked for milking cows in years past. Tears pressed forward as a smile burst forth. I pictured Jim giving his signature nod and hand raise to the farmer. I couldn't stop myself, I had to imitate him. I chuckled softly to myself as the farmer returned the nod and hand raise.

As cars started to file onto my front lawn at home, we let the kids out. Rene and I had a few minutes to talk. I was getting the impression that he thought we were handling this better than he thought we would be.

"Rene, Jim always said, 'God has blessed me with fifty-four great years. I have been blessed beyond what I could have imagined. I have no regrets.' Not only that but what kind of wife would I be if I was wanting him back all the time? Yes, I miss him. I miss him very much," I said as tears started to rise. Then, taking a deep breath I continued, "As his wife, I should want the best for him. What could be better than heaven? Why would I want him back here in this broken world with pain and sorrow? Jim prepared us. He was accepting of his death and that makes it easier for the rest of us to accept his death." I could see him thinking. We talked a bit more before one of the kids came to ask me if they could start cutting the cake. I sent him my apologies saying I would like to continue this conversation later and he agreed. We then went to join the growing crowd of about seventy-five people in the front yard for cake and coffee. Later we would share in the chili dinner I had simmering in the massive roasting pan.

Ramblings

I AM A widow…

That can't be right. It seems so odd to my ears. That's not me. Sometimes it feels like the time I had with him was only a dream, a vivid dream. But then I look around and see my kids and grandkids. They are part of that "dream," but they are still here.

Sometimes if I close my eyes, I can feel him. I can feel the stubble of his beard. I can run my thumb over his full lips. I can see his laugh lines in the corners of his eyes, I can feel my heart beat faster as I look into his smoky eyes, those rarely seen serious eyes. The eyes that looked into my heart and whispered, "I love you, Joanne." I feel very loved, cherished, and cared for. I miss laying with my back to him at night, with his arms wrapped around me holding me close. Is that why I wake up laying across the bed sideways? Am I searching for him in my sleep? Those feelings and memories are so precious to me. I don't want to forget them. I was so blessed to have Jim in my life.

I also feel we were blessed by the way things happened. We could say goodbye. Jim helped us mourn. He helped by holding me when I was mad about things we were losing. We cried together. Yet by the end, he was not himself. I don't know how to explain it. He just was not the same.

God is looking out for me. But who am I now without Jim? I am missing my other half, feeling incomplete. Where do I belong?

Six months without Jim. Yes, I can say his name. Yes, I love it when you mention his name or tell me stories about your memories of him. So do my kids. It's a gift. These stories might bring tears to our eyes, but that is okay, as it just means we are healing. There is no time limit on this healing and the length is different for each person. Just remember it can't be rushed and we *have* to go through it. Talking to other widows and widowers I have found out that you have to learn to live with it, cope with it and survive it. As time goes by, we will get better at it. The anger will soften, the tears will abate, and the future will be brighter than it is today. But we will never be cured, not even those who remarry, I'm told.

What I can tell you is that those emotional ambushes are really hard. They come out of nowhere. I would look across the living room and see his truck out the window. And then it happened. I had to move it to the other driveway, which was not visible from inside the house all day. In the grocery store, I would see Jim's favourite food. And then it happened. It didn't happen last week when I saw it, but today it did. On the rare occasion it happens when I see a woman with her arms tight around her man as they are on their touring motorcycle. Sometimes when a grandchild's comical antics make you want to share with Jim. Like when I saw a picture of my granddaughter Aria, with a big smile on her face, holding one of Papa's chickens. Another time I went, smiling, to the front counter to register for a conference. They handed me my nametag. I looked down and read "Ms. Schreud-ers." Then it happened. The friend who I came with looked over at me, asking if I was okay, not understanding what could have triggered my glassy eyes and quiver-ing chin, as I had been doing so well. Showing her the nametag, she understood and leaned in for a quick hug. And to her credit, we went on after she gave me a moment to regroup, as if it had just been a bump in the road. Another dear friend sent a beautiful encouragement card. "We miss Jim. We miss seeing you together." Then it happened. One Sunday, a Premier John Deere truck pulled into the church parking lot right before me. I didn't know if I would make it into the building. Then when I met my new precious granddaughter, the girl we had prayed for together, my daughter-in-law graciously brought Jim into the conversation, making the moment all that more special as we cried together. Those emotional ambushes sure play havoc on my life.

The best way I can think to explain what a widow is going through, is to think of those times when your spouse looks across the room at you and smiles. Or when you see that look in their eyes and you know what they are thinking. The way they touch you, say your name, joke with you. It goes on, all the things you share with *only* your spouse, no one else. These are all treasures, so rare and beautiful. Now I'm left with a lump of buried treasure sealed in its own tomb. Think about it for a minute. You will *never* get any of that back, *never*. You have to go on without it. That other part of you, that big, beautiful part, is gone. *Forever*!

Conversations may be difficult for you, but they are even harder for those of us who are grieving. Not only the spouse, but also the children. People seem to forget the children. Please don't go up to the children and ask how their parent is. Ask how *they* are. Maybe you hesitate because you know that, "I'm okay," really isn't an okay. And you are right, we are hurting. So why not instead of saying, "How are you?" you try, "What have you been doing?" That is a way that the conversation can continue more smoothly, and not stop awkwardly and abruptly.

We, those who grieve, want you to know that "What do you need?" is not helpful. We do not know what we need because we are in a fog of grief, and we cannot think clearly most of the time. Which makes us feel even worse for not being able to answer your vague question. What would be helpful is if you would take something specific off our plate. Ask with the intention to be helpful. If you want to help, offer clear and specific things. For example, "Is your freezer full of meals?" "Would you like a meal?" or "Can I shovel your driveway or mow your lawn for you?" or "Can I drive your kids somewhere for you?" "Can I take you out for coffee/lunch?" Any of which might get a "Not right now." Just remember that it might just be a really bad day. Just ask again later. Follow through.

Things have been done a certain way. The way to Jim's liking. I am learning he trained me well. He led, and I followed. I find myself trying to figure out this thought in my head, but it is very foggy. I want to see it clearly, but I can't. I will be doing something, and it will make me think of Jim. "I wonder what he would do?" "I wonder what he would think." But it doesn't matter. That's the part I get stuck on. It doesn't matter. I want it to matter, but it really doesn't. I get stuck there. I can't seem to move past that. How can his life not matter? He is a part of me. Things I do are because of him. But it doesn't matter, he is not here. If I do something different, not his way, that's okay.

Think about it

We can rest in this unknown future, knowing God walks with us. He is not only here today walking with us, but He is also already in our future. He is there preparing the way for us. We truly have nothing to fear. Walk with Him today. *"The Lord himself goes before you and will be with you; he will never leave you nor forsake you. Do not be afraid; do not be discouraged"* (Deuteronomy 31:8).

Reflections

HERE I STAND, a year after Jim's passing. Do I want to move on without Jim? No, definitely not. Can I move on? Yes, because I know God walks with me. I know He does, for He tells me in His word, the Bible. One such place is in Isaiah 43:1–3,

> *But now, this is what the Lord says – he who created you, O Jacob, he who formed you, O Israel: "Fear not, for I have redeemed you; I have summoned you by name; you are mine. When you pass through the waters, I will be with you; and when you pass through the rivers, they will not sweep over you. When you walk through the fire, you will not be burned; the flames will not set you ablaze. For I am the Lord, your God, the Holy One of Israel, your Savior.*

I thought I had an idea of what it would be like to live without Jim. But I honestly didn't know; I didn't have the faintest idea. Over the past year, I have slowly compiled a list of things I have lost. The list includes tangible things like my companion, mechanic, lumberjack, chimney sweep, dead mouse disposer, and gift giver. Someone to take care of me and do the chores when I'm sick. My entertainer, adventurer, breadwinner, encourager, and the one who kept me generous. But some losses were not as tangible. Someone who made those difficult decisions for me. Someone to blame when the decision was wrong—hee hee. Someone to tell me to stop snacking when I'm nervous. Someone to remind me I'm beautiful just the way I am. Someone who shared my dreams of the future. Someone to sit with and just "be" (without words). My hugger—the only arms that understood me and whose embrace could comfort me. My encourager, my shoulder to cry on, my bed warmer on cold winter nights, my lover, the one who could melt me with a look, my *best* friend.

As I look at this list of words, it doesn't touch the tip of how I feel. I can't explain it. Even if I could, it would not be the same for someone else. We all grieve differently. While those of us who grieve are hurting inside, we often think we must hide the tears from all of you around us. It is so much work. Putting on a happy face is exhausting. I genuinely ask that you encourage our tears. It's God's way of letting us wash some of that pain away, healing us.

God has led me to different things to help in the healing. I am very aware that I can only get through each day with the power God gives me through his Holy Spirit. Reading God's word, the Bible, or doing a devotional, is very challenging during these days, but the reassurances are very encouraging. Church is also a hard place to be for those of us who grieve. Like a child who gets hurt and can be brave until they see a parent; then they break down and weep. So is it for us who have lost a loved one when we enter into God's presence. The music is therapy to our souls, reaching down and bringing the tears to the surface, spilling over as we climb into God's comforting lap.

A book that helped me was *Widow to Widow: Thoughtful, Practical Ideas for Rebuilding Your Life*[13] by Genevieve Davis Ginsburg. By reading it I learned how others dealt with grief. I read of other people's stories, which helped me to not feel so alone, but instead to feel understood. They wrote about going through your husband's things, something each widow *needs* to do on their own; you should not do it for them as this step will help with the grieving. But they also suggested we have someone there when we do, someone who will sit there and listen to our stories as we go through their things. This should not be someone who will take over the process, which may cause regret later. There were also tips on taking over some of your husband's responsibilities, such as keeping up the house repairs or making large purchases. It was good to hear stories of others who have walked this walk, not only in a book, but in person.

I also signed up for the GriefShare[14] daily devotional emails. I found them very helpful. They always turned me back to trusting in God and His good and perfect plan. Before Christmas, I went to a GriefShare "Surviving the Holidays" workshop that a local church was hosting. I got great tips on how to make it through that hard season. I learned that driving myself to functions was a good idea, so I could leave when it got too hard. Also, making arrangements beforehand to possibly back out of an invitation last minute was okay. The material also suggested that helping others would be helpful to me. This was a way of taking the focus off myself and assisting

---

[13] Genevieve Davis Ginsburg, *Widow to Widow: Thoughtful, Practical Ideas for Rebuilding Your Life* (Boston: DaCapo Lifelong Books, 2004).

[14] "How to Heal from Grief," GriefShare, https://www.griefshare.org/healing.

others, making my life meaningful again. On the flip side, I also needed to find time to be silent—to listen to God and trust Him—and not be too busy. This was a hard thing for me to do, finding the balance between rest and being active.

Later in my grief journey, I slowly worked through a 90-day devotional book *Grieving God's Way: The Path to Lasting Hope and Healing* by Margaret Brownley.[15] This book was a breath of fresh air that I probably couldn't have read earlier in this journey. But now I was ready to give some effort to find where I belonged on this new path. Each day there was a small thing for me to do, which encouraged me to find that little bit of joy in life again.

Looking back to being nineteen and newly married, having left my father's house to start a home with Jim, I remember those exciting and scary times. But it was a time to create a new chapter in my life. Now with Jim gone, it feels like that chapter has ended. Putting the "J" charm on the end of my charm bracelet confirmed this.

Now I must start a new chapter. I must put one foot in front of the other. My life, as far as I can see, is not over. If I do the math, another lifetime with Jim will bring me to my mid-eighties and like Jim, I want to do it well. Looking back doesn't look like many years, but looking ahead does. How does God want me to use the future?

So, you might ask, "Are you ready to get on with your life?" It does not work like that. Jim has not left me or my thoughts. *"For this reason a man will leave his father and mother and be united to his wife, and they will become one flesh"* (Genesis 2:24). This passage has taken on yet another meaning. We are one flesh. A physical part of me is now in heaven.

I now ask myself daily, "What would Jim do?" And I here myself answer, "Jim would like this" or "He wouldn't like that!" He *is* part of me. We are one. I have even noticed the little things, like turning the front porch light on at night. He always did that. Why? I don't know why, but I find myself doing it now. It drives me crazy trying to remember to turn it on or off. So, why do it? I know it doesn't make sense, but it's only because he did it. (He would laugh if he knew he was still under my skin, irritating me in these small ways.)

As I talked with others who had lost a spouse years earlier, I learned that they also think of them daily. We will never "get over" them or get to the other side of grief. It doesn't work like that. Grief is always there; you learn to live with it, and it gets easier to manage daily. They are never gone.

It is hard to be a mom of a large, grieving family. Each of them processes it differently. Each of them hurts in their own way, and as their mom, I want to fix it and take the hurt away. But I know I can't. They, like me, need to work through their grief

---

[15] Margaret Brownley, *Grieving God's Way: The Path to Lasting Hope and Healing* (Nashville: Thomas Nelson, 2012).

independently. Only they can do it. I am here to listen, day or night. Some days it feels like this is all I do, which is okay. I love them dearly and want them to all be okay.

My kids who still live at home are what got me out of bed in the mornings. They helped me process other things that were happening around me. I do not know how seniors do it alone. I urge you to go to those widows and widowers and help them find reasons to carry on through life. Even knowing that you are coming to visit will help them get out of bed and get dressed in the morning. Short visits are all they need, probably all they can handle. Take your conversation cues from the grieving person and remember that silence is okay. Caring enough to come is huge for us. It is okay, and even welcome, to talk about the person who has passed. Name them by name. I cannot stress how much of a blessing it is to hear how our loved one impacted other people's lives. Instead of asking how we are feeling, ask what we are doing to keep busy. Practical help like mowing their lawn, feeding the dog, or offering to do some maintenance around their house can go a long way.

I have had kids say, "You can't be alone, mom. You will be too sad and lonely." But with my large family, I know I need those alone times. I sometimes need to have a good cry with no one around. With help from good friends who have surrounded me, I'm learning to take time for myself. In the meantime, I strive to follow God's leading. One way is by writing this book. By writing, I have been able to process what has happened. While it was happening, we were going through the motions. While writing, I could cry many tears or laugh out loud, recalling our times together. Letting those tears run down my cheeks helped me go out in public as a stronger person. On the days I didn't write, I found it more challenging to be in public. The tears just piled up behind my eyes, ready to overflow at any minute. The writing was therapy for me. I also found it surprising that I could be writing and crying but then turn around to listen to one of my children's stories and genuinely laugh with them. God is so good.

Jim had said, "I wish I could talk to someone who has been through this, but they are all gone." Even though he couldn't talk with others who went before him, he boldly took each day as it came, never choosing to be a victim. He chose God! The God that gave him the strength to go through those hard days. A God who helped him do it well.

Remember, death is just a door; Jesus is the way through this door to a life without pain and suffering. Knowing that death is part of life, I want to encourage you to talk about it and prepare for it with those around you. This was so helpful for all of us who were left behind. My hope and prayer are that our story may give you *hope*. The same hope that Jim had in a beautiful heavenly home that awaited him. A home that is far greater than anything we can ever imagine.

But in the meantime, God still has work for you and me to do here on this earth. So, I encourage you to step one foot in front of the other with me, in faith, to be used by God in this time.

> I pray that out of his glorious riches he may strengthen you with power through his Spirit in your inner being, so that Christ may dwell in your hearts though faith. And I pray that you, being rooted and established in love, may have power, together with all the saints, to grasp how wide and long and high and deep is the love of Christ, and to know this love that surpasses knowledge – that you may be filled to the measure of all the fullness of God. Now to him who is able to do immeasurably more than all we ask or imagine, according to his power that is at work within us, to him be glory in the church and in Christ Jesus throughout all generations, for ever and ever! Amen. (Ephesians 3: 16–21)

About the Author

JOANNE SCHREUDERS IS a Christian author, speaker, widow, and retired homeschool mom of ten with a growing number of grandchildren. She has a heart for helping others as they walk this journey of life.

SECURING YOUR LEGACY: TIPS ON DOING IT WELL
Joanne is excited to speak on the topic of "Securing Your Legacy: Tips on Doing It Well."

CONNECT WITH HER FOR MORE INFORMATION:
Facebook: facebook.com/joanne.schreuders
Instagram: @joanneschreuders

Also by Joanne Schreuders

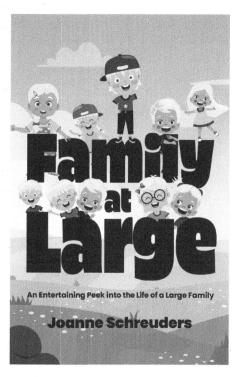

An Entertaining Peek into the Life of a Large Family

Joanne Schreuders

ISBN: 978-1-4866-2550-5

HAVE YOU EVER wondered what it would be like to parent a large family? Or does the idea of having "all those kids" scare you? Joanne Schreuders, a homeschooling mother of ten, shares an inside look at her life raising a large family. Between the covers of this book, you'll find humorous tales of flannel bunnies, bookstores, and Christmas turkeys, along with a balance of life tips and Joanne's thoughts on being a mother. Some say mothers of large families are *Super Moms,* but Joanne shares a different take on this unique lifestyle, one that requires a *Super God*!